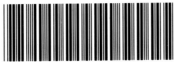

CURRENT CLINICAL UROLOGY

ERIC A. KLEIN, MD, SERIES EDITOR
PROFESSOR OF SURGERY
CLEVELAND CLINIC LERNER COLLEGE OF MEDICINE
SECTION OF UROLOGIC ONCOLOGY
GLICKMAN UROLOGICAL AND KIDNEY INSTITUTE
CLEVELAND, OH

For further volumes:
http://www.springer.com/series/7635

Philippe E. Spiess

Editor

Penile Cancer

Diagnosis and Treatment

Foreword by Francesco Montorsi

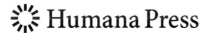 Humana Press

Editor
Philippe E. Spiess, MD, MS
Department of Genitourinary Oncology
Moffitt Cancer Center
Tampa, FL, USA

ISBN 978-1-62703-366-4   ISBN 978-1-62703-367-1 (eBook)
DOI 10.1007/978-1-62703-367-1
Springer New York Heidelberg Dordrecht London

Library of Congress Control Number: 2013933237

Printed on acid-free paper

Humana Press is a brand of Springer
Springer is part of Springer Science+Business Media (www.springer.com)

Foreword

The present book dedicated to the significant advances made in the field of penile cancer has been edited by Dr. Philippe E. Spiess, and an emphasis has been placed on highlighting the important diagnostic and therapeutic considerations in the management of this highly aggressive tumor phenotype. Thought leaders in the field of penile cancer research and clinical care have contributed to this effort and convey important treatment considerations in the management of this malignancy. Afflicted patients have traditionally undergone mutilating surgery, with life-altering implications, but as highlighted in this text, penile sparing surgical approaches can be offered to a select subset of patients, with excellent functional outcomes without compromising oncological efficacy. Similarly, minimally invasive surgical approaches to the inguinal lymph nodes in patients not exhibiting palpable inguinal lymphadenopathy encompass dynamic sentinel lymph node biopsy techniques and laparoendoscopic (pure or robotic) inguinal lymph node dissection. Lastly, patients with bulky/locally advanced inguinal lymph node metastases have traditionally been faced with a dismal prognosis (typically 5 year survival rates ranging between 10 and 30 %); however, exciting advancements using a multimodal approach of upfront systemic chemotherapy followed by consolidative surgical resection are currently redefining our treatment paradigm.

It is quite evident that great strides have been made in the management of penile cancer in the past decade, but unfortunately it remains that this malignancy constitutes a highly aggressive tumor histology particularly in those with advanced disease. The role of human papilloma virus immunization in patient populations at increased risk of this malignancy is an active area of socio-epidemiological research. Similarly, the role of novel diagnostic modalities such as PET/CT and of targeted therapies aimed at the EGFR pathway particularly in penile cancer patients, in whom it is strongly overexpressed, is of significant clinical interest and may truly revolutionize our therapeutic approach to advanced penile cancer. Unquestionably, the field of penile cancer fosters a bright horizon, which is a testament of the significant

contributions made to both clinical and translational research. I encourage
all of you caring for penile cancer patients to read this book, as it will likely
impact your views and treatment approach to this cancer type for the many
years to come.

Francesco Montorsi, MD
Professor of Urology, Milan, Italy
University Vita-Salute San Rafaelle
Editor-in-Chief, **European Urology**

Contents

Contributors

Hussain M. Alnajjar, M.B.B.S., B.Sc. (Med Sci.), M.R.C.S. Department of Urology, St. George's Hospital, London, UK

Matthew Biagioli, M.D., M.S. Department of Radiation Oncology, H. Lee Moffitt Cancer Center, Tampa, FL, USA

Rafael Clavijo, M.D. Department of Urology, Hospital de San Jose, Bogota, Colombia

Juanita Crook, M.D. Department of Radiation Oncology, British Columbia Cancer Agency, Kelowna, BC, Canada

Rosa S. Djajadiningrat, M.D. Department of Urologic Oncology, Antoni van Leeuwenhoek Hospital, The Netherlands Cancer Institute, Amsterdam, The Netherlands

Cesar E. Ercole, M.D. Department of Urology, University of South Florida, Tampa, FL, USA

Adam S. Feldman, M.D., M.P.H. Department of Urology, Massachusetts General Hospital, Boston, MA, USA

O.W. Hakenberg, M.D., Ph.D. Department of Urology, University of Rostock, Rostock, Germany

Paul K. Hegarty, M.B.,B.Ch., B.A.O., F.R.C.S.I., F.R.C.S. (Urol), M.Med. Sc., M.Ch., M.B.A. (Life Sciences) Department of Urology, Guy's and St Thomas' NHS Foundation Trust, London, UK

Simon Horenblas, M.D., Ph.D. Department of Urologic Oncology, Antoni van Leeuwenhoek Hospital, The Netherlands Cancer Institute, Amsterdam, The Netherlands

Brant A. Inman, M.D., M.S. Division of Urology, Department of Surgery, Duke University Medical Center, Durham, NC, USA

Michael W. Kattan, Ph.D. Department of Quantitative Health Sciences, Cleveland Clinic, Cleveland, OH, USA

W. Scott McDougal, M.D. Department of Urology, Massachusetts General Hospital, Boston, MA, USA

Lance C. Pagliaro, M.D. Department of Genitourinary Medical Oncology, The University of Texas MD Anderson Cancer Center, Houston, TX, USA

Curtis A. Pettaway, M.D. Department of Urology, University of Texas M.D. Anderson Cancer Center, Houston, TX, USA

C. Protzel, M.D., Ph.D. Department of Urology, University of Rostock, Rostock, Germany

Priya Rao, M.B.B.S., M.D. Department of Pathology, The University of Texas M.D. Anderson Cancer Center, Houston, TX, USA

Rafael Sanchez-Salas, M.D. Department of Urology, Institut Mutualiste Monsouris, Paris, France

Majid Shabbir, F.R.C.S. (Urol) Department of Urology, St. George's Hospital, London, UK

René Sotelo, M.D. Department of Urology, Instituto Médico La Floresta, Caracas, Venezuela

Philippe E. Spiess, M.D., M.S. Department of Genitourinary Oncology, Moffitt Cancer Center, Tampa, FL, USA

Suzanne B. Stewart, M.D. Division of Urology, Department of Surgery, Duke University Medical Center, Durham, NC, USA

Pheroze Tamboli, M.B.B.S. Department of Pathology, The University of Texas M.D. Anderson Cancer Center, Houston, TX, USA

Nicholas A. Watkin, M.Ch., F.R.C.S. (Urol) Department of Urology, St. George's Hospital, London, UK

Epidemiology and Risk Factors for Penile Cancer

Paul K. Hegarty

Epidemiology

The incidence of penile cancer varies greatly globally. The incidence in the Western world is in the range of 0.3–1/100,000 males. In the USA the incidence is 0.81 per 100,000 men [1, 2], of which 40% of cases are associated with HPV carriage [3, 4]. The rate in Paraguay is 4.2 per 100,000 according to the International Agency for Research on Cancer (IARC) [5]. Within malignancies its incidence ranges from <0.5% of all male cancers in the USA to 10–20% in parts of South America, Asia and Africa [6]. The highest cumulative rate of 1% before age 75 is seen in parts of Uganda, whereas the lowest cumulative rate is 300 times less amongst Israeli Jews. Areas with higher incidences have a greater proportion of young men with penile cancer [7]. The incidence increases with age. The age distribution among patients from one series of consecutive patients in a superregional referral unit in the UK is represented in Fig. 1.1.

P.K. Hegarty, M.B. B.Ch., B.A.O., F.R.C.S.I., F.R.C.S. (Urol), M. Med Sc., M.Ch., M.B.A. (Life Sciences) (✉)
Department of Urology, Guy's and St Thomas' NHS Foundation Trust, Great Maze Pond,
London SE1 9RT, UK
e-mail: paulhegarty@gstt.nhs.uk

Risk Factors in the Pathogenesis of Penile Cancer

The exact pathway leading to penile carcinogenesis has yet to be clarified, but several contributing factors have been identified, some of which are corroborated by molecular biology, others not.

Human Papilloma Virus

Human papilloma virus (HPV) is an uncoated double chain DNA-virus. It comes from the family of the papova viruses and it is made up of two capsids (L1 and L2). Thus far there are at least 100 known variants. These have been classified by Munoz [9] according to their oncogenic potential (Table 1.1). HPV is implicated in the pathogenesis of several cancers, most notably cervical cancer in women. Depending on the size of the cohort and techniques HPV is found in about 50% of cases of penile cancer [10–12]. However, a recent Swedish study demonstrated 70% HPV positivity out of 216 cases of penile cancer [13], with 80.8% of invasive cases being HPV positive. A systematic review examined the prevalence of HPV in 1,266 cases of penile cancer from 30 studies [14]. The mean prevalence of HPV was 47.9% within a range of 14.6–100%. Variations in reported incidences may reflect technical issues with demonstrating the presence of HPV or on the prevalence of certain histological subtypes within the cohort,

P.E. Spiess (ed.), *Penile Cancer: Diagnosis and Treatment*, Current Clinical Urology,
DOI 10.1007/978-1-62703-367-1_1, © Springer Science+Business Media New York 2013

Fig. 1.1 Age at presentation among 100 consecutive cases in a UK centre [8]

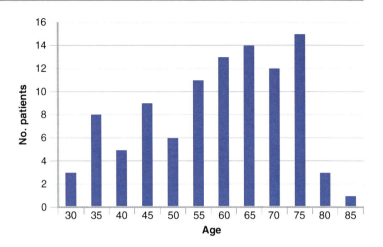

Table 1.1 HPV subtype associated with carcinogenesis (modified from Munoz [9])

Classification	HPV subtypes
High risk carcinogen	16,18,31,33,35,39,45,51,52,56,58, 58
Probable carcinogen	26,53,66,68,73,82
Low risk carcinogen	6,11,40,42,43,44,54,61,70,72, 81,CP6108

as basaloid and warty are more likely to be HPV positive than other subtypes [15]. The variation in incidence between high prevalence areas, e.g. Paraguay, and low prevalence, e.g. USA, does not appear to be explained for by HPV subtype carriage rate, as a retrospective histopathological study from the two countries has shown [16].

More than 100 subtypes of HPV have been described [17]. The predominant subtypes associated with carcinogenesis are 16 and 18.

The role of high risk HPV infection in penile cancer seems to be variable and is not clear. In contrast to healthy controls, the prevalence of HPV-infection differs markedly. In a North American case–control study, positive HPV-16 serology was found among 24% of cases and 12% of controls (odds ratio, 1.9; 95% CI, 1.2–3.2), at a tissue level 80% of penile cancer were positive for HPV DNA [18].

In similar study from Uganda, seropositivity to HPV-16, HPV-18 or HPV-45, the most common oncogenic types of HPV, was 46% among penile cancer cases and 12% among controls (odds ratio, 5.0; 95% CI, 1.4–17.2) [19]. How HPV impacts on the behaviour of penile cancer and how it influences prognosis has been investigated by several authors, with conflicting results. Gregoire et al. described a more aggressive vertical tumour growth and more likely poorly differentiated cancers in those positive for HPV [11]. Daling et al. also found an increased risk for invasive cancers with HPV-16 positive serology [18], whereas Wiener et al. and Bezerra et al. found no such correlation [20, 21].

Intracellular Activity of HPV

High risk HPV appears to act through its viral genes E6 and E7 which alter proliferation, apoptosis and differentiation through the retinoblastoma (Rb) and p53 tumour suppressor pathways. The protein product of E6 binds to p53 blocking its normal inhibitory function at the G1/S phase of the cell cycle. This leads to uncontrolled proliferation, decreased apoptosis and cellular dedifferentiation [22]. Invasive penile cancers that are negative for HPV tend to have mutant p53 as shown in a small cohort from Japan [23]. Mutant p53 predicts for lymph node positivity and mortality [24]. Thus, it would appear that perturbation of p53 is central to pathogenesis either through its mutation or inhibition. One of the proposed mechanisms of invasion of cancers is through epithelial-mesenchymal transition. Cell surface receptors change with the phenotypic flux between epithelial and mesenchymal states. In studying penile cancer invasion, Campos et al. demonstrated low E-cadherin is associated with the risk of lymph node metastasis [25]. The matrix metalloproteinase MMP-2 and MMP-9 have been studied in many solid cancers and are thought to be involved in the process of invasion of primary tumours into adjacent tissue [26]. In penile cancer, MMP-9 is associated with a greater risk of recurrent disease [25]. Greater detail of the current understanding of the molecular basis of penile cancer is described in a review by Muneer et al. [15].

Presence of Foreskin

Neonatal circumcision seems to be protective against penile cancer later in life. Countries whose males are for the most part circumcised as infants have exceedingly low rates of penile cancer [7]. Furthermore phimosis is more prevalent among patients presenting with penile cancer. Therefore, the inner preputial environment is likely to be an important factor. It would appear that circumcision can help prevention of acquisition/maintenance of carcinogenic HPV subtypes. In a cohort of 379 mostly heterosexual men in Hawaii, the prevalence of HPV on the glans/coronal sulcus was 46% among uncircumcised men as compared to 29% of circumcised men [1]. However, the magnitude of protective effect of neonatal circumcision appears to be greater than just HPV prevention. In addition, neonatal rather than teenage circumcision is also more protective which suggests that the prepubertal environment is somehow involved in the pathogenesis of penile cancer. It may be that phimosis and balanoposthitis are involved in the pathogenesis of penile cancer. The reduced rate of penile cancer may be mainly explained by the prevention of phimosis/balanoposthitis, smegma retention, and lichen sclerosus.

Phimosis

The term phimosis originates from the Greek word for muzzle (φιμος) denoting unretractable foreskin. In the first years of life, it is physiological and can persist into teenage years [27, 28]. Phimosis can also be acquired. The most commonly seen acquired phimoses are with chronic inflammation, balanoposthitis, lichen sclerosus, following trauma or associated with diabetes. Among uncircumcised males the incidence of phimosis ranges between 8 and 23% [29]. The observed differences are likely due to different regions studied, age at diagnosis and the varying definitions of phimosis.

A population based case–control study reported by Tseng et al. included 100 matched case–control pairs in Los Angeles County [30]. There was a strong association between phimosis and penile invasive cancer. They described an inverse correlation between penile cancer and neonatal circumcision; however, the correlation was considerably weakened when the analysis was restricted to subjects with no history of phimosis. The study concluded that the protective effect of neonatal circumcision appeared to be largely mediated through the prevention of phimosis.

Infection

Balanitis and posthitis are the respective inflammations of the glans and prepuce. A case–control study from Sweden was reported by Dillner [31]. Among 244 patients, the authors found that 45% of patients had at least one episode of balanitis, compared with 8% of controls. Men with diabetes are a specifically high risk group, in whom balanitis occurs in 35%.

Hygiene

There is not much evidence of the association between hygiene and penile cancer. In a study of cervical cancer in Punjab, India where it is the most common malignancy in females, Nagpal et al. postulated "that a common carcinogenic agent, either a virus or a biochemical (smegmatic) factor, may be responsible for the high incidence of carcinoma of the penis in males and carcinoma of the cervix in females" [32]. However, van Howe and Hodges studied the current evidence of any carcinogenic properties of smegma. They found that there was no scientific justification to support the hypothesis that smegma is carcinogenic [33].

A cross sectional study by O'Farrell postulates a potential link between circumcision and penile hygiene. Poor genital hygiene behaviour was seen more commonly among uncircumcised (26%) men than among circumcised (4%). Of the circumcised group, 37% washed more than once a day, as compared to 19% of the uncircumcised cohort [34].

Frisch et al. studied the long term changes in the incidence of penile cancer in an uncircumcised population from Denmark between 1943 and 1990. They indicated that the decrease in incidence of penile cancer in Denmark may be as a result of better penile hygiene, from improvements in sanitary installations in that country [35]. Denmark probably represents the first country to institute public health measures to prevent occupational related cancer. In the nineteenth century, compulsory daily baths reduced the incidence of squamous cancer of the scrotum among chimney sweeps [36].

Zoophilia

A case-controlled study from Brazil interviewed nearly 500 men regarding their personal and sexual practices; 118 had penile cancer and 374 did not [37]. Univariate and multivariate analyses were performed. The study found 44.9% of men with penile cancer reported having had sex with animals, as compared to 31.6% among those without penile cancer. Subjects who admitted to having sex with animals were also more likely to have had sexually transmitted infection, to have engaged in sex with prostitutes and to have had more than ten partners. Thus, zoophilia may be an indicator of other high risk sexual behaviours rather than a cause in itself of penile cancer. On multivariate analysis, within this study, phimosis, premalignant lesions, smoking and zoophilia were all identified as risk factors for penile cancer.

PUVA Treatment

Psoralen and long-wave ultraviolet radiation (PUVA) is used in the treatment of psoriasis. A case of squamous cell cancer of the penis following such treatment was reported by Tam et al. [38]. A prospective series reported by Stern reported on 892 men over a 12-year follow-up period. When patients were treated with high levels of oral methoxsalen (8-methoxypsoralen) and ultraviolet A photochemotherapy (PUVA), the incidence of genital cancer was 286 times higher than the general population. There was a strong dose dependent relationship with the risk of genital cancers [39]. This cohort has now been followed for 30 years [40]. Squamous cell cancer risk was far higher than that of basal cell cancer. PUVA patients should be advised to carefully shield the genitalia and observe skin changes, especially after high levels of PUVA therapy.

Socioeconomic Factors

The protective effect of neonatal circumcision from a cancer that presents several decades later may imply that other environmental factors are involved in the pathogenesis of this malignancy. In the USA, the relationship between social factors and penile cancer has been reported [41]. This study showed that lack of medical insurance was associated with late presentation and lymph node metastasis. Forty-five percent of men in this study were lost to follow-up, although lack of insurance was not a risk factor for this. Excessive consumption of alcohol is associated with squamous cell cancers elsewhere in the body. Its association with penile cancer however is not clear cut. One theory on its involvement in pathogenesis is that a cirrhotic liver is less efficient at removing carcinogens from the circulation. Alcohol abuse may indicate self-neglect that can delay presentation and reduce an individual's ability to cope with the diagnosis and engage in treatment and follow-up. In any case, noting the alcohol habits is important as it may impact men perioperatively and their ability to tolerate chemotherapy.

Smoking

In epidemiological studies, smoking is seen to be consistently associated to penile cancer. A review by Dillner et al. identified a clear association between smoking and penile cancer that was not explained by the presence of other risk factors such as sexual history and phimosis [31]. There is a significant association between smoking or chewing tobacco and penile carcinoma, as described by Harish and Ravi [42]. They looked at over 500 men with penile cancer and age matched controls. Multivariate analysis showed a significant association, which was reinforced by a demonstrable dose dependent relationship. Daling et al. calculated an OR for penile cancer of 2.3 according to the active smoking status. Interestingly the man's HPV-status did not change the increased OR for smokers in contrast to non-smokers. In particular, current smokers had a considerable increase OR 4.5 for invasive cancer, which was a noticeable difference from the more moderate increased risk for former smokers [18]. Thus, smoking cessation is essential to primary prevention. The importance of tobacco avoidance must be emphasised with men who have premalignant skin conditions.

Premalignant Dermatoses

There is several skin conditions found in association with penile cancer. These are covered in Chap. 3. Secondary prevention may be used to screen patients with these lesions for penile cancer. However, some of the more common conditions such as balanitis xerotica obliterans/lichen sclerosis may make it impractical to have patients under review in a specialised clinic. A programme of self-examination and facilitation of access to specialised care may be a more sensible approach.

Preventative Strategies

Primary prevention has clear advantages; however, there is a dearth of literature on the topic concerning penile cancer. Based on our understanding of the pathophysiologic basis of penile

Table 1.2 Possible risk factors for penile and risk reduction strategies [43]

Risk factors for the development of penile cancer	Preventative measures
HPV infections	HPV-vaccination, condom use
Phimosis	Circumcision
Chronic balanoposthitis	Therapy of genital inflammation
Smoking	Smoking prevention/cessation
Smegma retention/poor hygiene	Hygiene education
Penile oral sex	Sexual education
Lifetime number of female sex partners	
Alcohol excess	Alcohol abstinence
Urethral stricture	Secondary prevention/early detection
PUVA therapy	

cancer, there are a number of options for primary prevention of penile cancer. These include circumcision, HPV prevention, smoking cessation and possibly hygienic measures (Table 1.2).

Rationale for HPV Vaccination

There is a clear association between HPV and penile cancer, although the natural history and treatment of HPV is confined to small series, most of which are retrospective.

The relationship between HPV-infection and subsequent development of cervical cancer is well established. Approval studies for HPV-vaccines included boys between 9 and 15 years of age. Following vaccination, they had a sero-conversion rate comparable to girls. In fact the anti HPV-immunoreaction was higher among boys and girls than in women. The protective effect from HPV infection is confident for 5 years after vaccination. Data in longer term is not currently available, so it is only an assumption at present that male vaccination could prevent development of HPV associated penile cancer. If HPV vaccination is recommended it should be given prior to sexual debut. Candidates should be aware that HPV vaccination may reduce but not eliminate the risk of penile cancer. Two vaccines

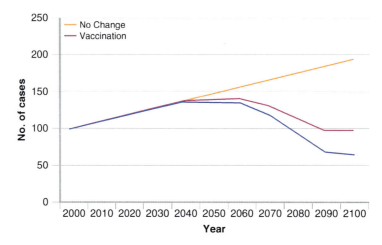

Fig. 1.2 Projected number of cases of penile cancer in the one region of the UK, based purely on demographics (no change), a programme of HPV vaccination or circumcision

have been brought to market. *Cervarix* is a bivalent vaccine targeting HPV-16 and -18; *Gardasil* is a quadrivalent vaccine which targets HPV-6, -11, -16 and -18. As HPV-16 and -18 are most commonly associated with cervical cancer, vaccination could prevent nearly 70% of all cervical cancers. Thus, vaccination is restricted to countries with predominantly HPV-16 and HPV-18 infections. The incidence of penile cancer may also be impacted by population-wide vaccination programmes. If females only are vaccinated then men may benefit from reduced risk of infection from women. However, even for the sake of preventing cervical cancer only, there may be benefit to vaccinating males [44]. Pharmacoeconomic modelling can provide the rationale for a vaccination programme for both males and females. Thus, a dynamic model with the aim of reducing the risk of cervical cancer suggested the most effective programme would be to use the quadrivalent HPV vaccine to boys and girls aged 12, combined with catch-up vaccination of both sexes between 12 and 24 [45].

In particular if uptake among the female population is poor, e.g. 50% of targeted age groups, then the cost–benefit ratio tends to favour inclusion of males in the programme. Depending on HPV prevalence and its subtype, it can be expected that HPV vaccination of males would reduce the incidence of penile cancer by about 50%. The lead-time to benefit would be several decades (Fig. 1.2).

Circumcision

It is estimated that globally 25% of men are circumcised [46]. Prior to 1999, the American Academy of Pediatrics used to recommend routine neonatal circumcision for health related reasons [47]. This was aimed at reducing the rate of infant urinary tract infection through avoidance of balanoposthitis and upper urinary tract infections, particularly in patients with vesicoureteric reflux. Circumcision as a measure to prevent penile cancer has been advocated by different authors, as the incidence of penile cancer is significantly lower in circumcised men compared to those who have not undergone circumcision.

The reduced rate of penile cancer is mainly explained by the effective reduction of phimosis/balanoposthitis, smegma retention and preventing cofactors such as HPV infection in comparison to non-circumcised men. In 1855, Hutchinson proposed that circumcision could prevent infection with syphilis [48]. A case–control study from several centres involving 1913 couples, men who were circumcised had an OR for HPV infection of 0.37, when corrected for potential confounding factors such as number of sexual partners.

There was an associated reduced risk of cervical cancer in the female partners of circumcised men [49]. Daling et al. reported a case–control study in the USA assessing the effect of childhood circumcision in preventing penile cancer later in life. They concluded that men who were not circumcised as a child had a 1.5-fold greater risk of subsequently developing penile cancer [18]. The argument in favour of circumcision has re-emerged due in part to the observed risk of reduction of 50–60% of contracting HIV infection in recent studies [50].

In the UK, circumcision is performed predominantly for medical reasons, as only 0.3% of boys are circumcised before the age of five [51]. Taking the data mentioned in Fig. 1.1 and projecting the changes in demographics by 2050, the number of cases will increase by 47%. A proposed programme of circumcising all males up to the age of 10 by the year 2015, with the presumption of reducing the risk of penile cancer by two-thirds will have no impact in the incidence for several decades as by 2050 men who are 55 years and older will have not benefited from the programme, leaving the projected incidence unchanged. The projected effect of HPV vaccination or circumcision is once again demonstrated in Fig. 1.2.

Thus, some authors describe circumcision as a biomedical imperative to reduce the risk of urinary tract infections, sexually transmitted disease, inflammatory conditions of the penis and penile cancer [29]. This is supported by Daling et al. who concluded that offering circumcision to boys may help prevent penile cancer by eliminating phimosis and avoiding co-factors of HPV infection [18]. However, the strategy remains controversial. Its benefit is likely to vary between countries. In the UK, where neonatal circumcision is not routine, disease-free survival for penile cancer in a contemporary series exceeds 90% [8]. As the incidence of cancer is about 1 per 100,000 males, this translates to circumcising about one million boys to prevent one death from penile cancer per year. However, areas of higher prevalence, such as in parts of Africa and South America, are the more sensible targets of such programmes, especially if combined with HIV preventative strategies.

Condom Use

Depending on the population it is estimated that about 50% of penile cancer is due to previous HPV infection. Prevention of HPV infection through the blocking transmission of HPV between sexual partners may lead to a long-term reduction in incidence of penile cancer. There is scant evidence on the effect of condom use for the prevention of HPV infection. Wen et al. described a retrospective case–control study of nearly 1,000 patients with HPV. They demonstrated a protective effect of condom use in patients with genital warts. In males and females, there was an independently associated increased risk of acquisition of genital warts if condoms were not used, whereas unfailing condom use was shown to be associated with a decreased risk of acquiring genital warts [52].

A follow up study of 82 female students in a university setting showed that for newly sexually active women, reliable condom use by male partners seemed to reduce the risk of HPV infection of cervix and genitals [53]. Furthermore when couples reported 100% condom use, there were no cervical squamous intraepithelial lesions observed when compared to couples who did not use condoms.

A randomised trial of heterosexual couples was reported in which the female had cervical intraepithelial neoplasia and her male partner had HPV associated flat lesions of the penis [54]. Couples were then randomised for the use/not use of a condom. Men in the condom use group were seen to have a significantly reduced interval to regression of the flat lesion on the penis. It is thought this phenomenon is probably due to the blocking of repeated viral transmission between the sexual partners [55].

Conclusion

The great variation between incidences in penile cancer seems to be due to environmental factors. HPV accounts for about half of penile cancers, with intracellular pathways described. Unlike the more common cancers, the genomic changes of penile cancer have yet to be reported. The interaction of environmental carcinogens and the genome is likely to be fascinating and provide new targets for treatment. High risk areas should be the priority for preventative programmes, although it will take several decades for benefit to accrue. Despite such strategies it is likely that oncological services for penile cancer will be needed for the rest of this century.

References

1. Hernandez BY, Wilkens LR, Zhu X, McDuffie K, Thompson P, Shvetsov YB, et al. Circumcision and human papillomavirus infection in men: a site-specific comparison. J Infect Dis. 2008;197:787–94.
2. Barnholtz-Sloan JS, Maldonado JL, Pow-sang J, Giuliano AR. Incidence trends in primary malignant penile cancer. Urol Oncol. 2007;25:361–7. Erratum in: Urol Oncol 2008; 26: 112. Guiliano, Anna R [corrected to Giuliano, Anna R].
3. Heideman DA, Waterboer T, Pawlita M, Delis-van Diemen P, Nindl I, Leijte JA, et al. Human papillomavirus-16 is the predominant type etiologically involved in penile squamous cell carcinoma. J Clin Oncol. 2007;25:4550–6.
4. Maden C, Sherman KJ, Beckmann AM, Hislop TG, Teh CZ, Ashley RL, et al. History of circumcision, medical conditions, and sexual activity and risk of penile cancer. J Natl Cancer Inst. 1993;85:19–24.
5. Parkin DM, Muir CS. Cancer incidence in five continents. Comparability and quality of data. IARC Sci Publ. 1992;120:45–173.
6. Wabinga HR, Parkin DM, Wabwire-Mangen F, et al. Trends in cancer incidence in Kyadondo County, Uganda 1960–1997. Br J Cancer. 2000;82:1585–92.
7. Cubilla AL, Dillner J, Schelhammer PF, et al. Tumors of the penis. Malignant epithelial tumors. In: Eble JN, Sauter G, Epstein JI, Sesterhenn IA, editors. World Health Organization Classification of Tumors. Pathology and genetics. Tumors of the urinary system and male genital organs. Lyon: IARC Press; 2004. p. 281–90.
8. Hegarty PK, Kayes O, Freeman A, Christopher AN, Ralph DJ, Minhas S. A prospective study of 100 cases of penile cancer managed according to EAU guidelines. BJU Int. 2006;98:526–31.
9. Muñoz N, Bosch FX, de Sanjosé S, Herrero R, Castellsagué X, Shah KV, et al. Epidemiologic classification of human papillomavirus types associated with cervical cancer. N Engl J Med. 2003; 348:518–27.
10. Rubin MA, Kleter B, Zhou M, Ayala G, Cubilla AL, Quint WG, et al. Detection and typing of human papillomavirus DNA in penile carcinoma: evidence for multiple independent pathways of penile carcinogenesis. Am J Pathol. 2001;159:1211–8.
11. Gregoire L, Cubilla AL, Reuter VE, Haas GP, Lancaster WD. Preferential association of human papillomavirus with high-grade histologic variants of penile-invasive squamous cell carcinoma. J Natl Cancer Inst. 1995;87:1705–9.
12. Cubilla AL, Lloveras B, Alejo M, Clavero O, Chaux A, Kasamatsu E, et al. The basaloid cell is the best tissue marker for human papillomavirus in invasive penile squamous cell carcinoma: a study of 202 cases from Paraguay. Am J Surg Pathol. 2010;34:104–14.
13. Kirrander P, Kolaric A, Helenius G, Windahl T, Andrén O, Stark JR, et al. Human papillomavirus prevalence, distribution and correlation to histopathological parameters in a large Swedish cohort of men with penile carcinoma. BJU Int. 2011;108:355–9.
14. Backes DM, Kurman RJ, Pimenta JM, Smith JS. Systematic review of human papillomavirus prevalence in invasive penile cancer. Cancer Causes Control. 2009;20:449–57.
15. Muneer A, Kayes O, Ahmed HU, Arya M, Minhas S. Molecular prognostic factors in penile cancer. World J Urol. 2009;27:161–7.
16. Chaux A, Tamboli P, Lezcano C, Ro J, Ayala A, Cubilla AL. Comparison of subtypes of penile squamous cell carcinoma from high and low incidence geographical regions. Int J Surg Pathol. 2010; 18: 268–77.
17. Muñoz N, Castellsagué X, de González AB, Gissmann L. Chapter 1: HPV in the etiology of human cancer. Vaccine. 2006;24 Suppl 3:S3/1–S3/10.
18. Daling JR, Madeleine MM, Johnson LG, Schwartz SM, Shera KA, Wurscher MA, et al. Penile cancer: importance of circumcision, human papillomavirus and smoking in in situ and invasive disease. Int J Cancer. 2005;116:606.
19. Newton R, Bousarghin L, Ziegler J, Uganda Kaposi's Sarcoma Study Group. Human papillomaviruses and cancer in Uganda. Eur J Cancer Prev. 2004;2:113–8.
20. Wiener JS, Effert PJ, Humphrey PA, et al. Prevalence of human papillomavirus types 16 and 18 in squamous-cell carcinoma of the penis: a retrospective analysis of primary and metastatic lesions by differential polymerase chain reaction. Int J Cancer. 1992; 50: 694–701.
21. Bezerra AL, Lopes A, Santiago GH, et al. Human papillomavirus as a prognostic factor in carcinoma of the penis: analysis of 82 patients treated with amputation and bilateral lymphadenectomy. Cancer. 2001; 91:2315–21.
22. Couturier J, Sastre-Garau X, Schneider-Maunoury S, Labib A, Orth G. Integration of papillomavirus DNA near myc genes in genital carcinomas and its consequences for proto-oncogene expression. J Virol. 1991; 65:4534–8.
23. Yanagawa N, Osakabe M, Hayashi M, Tamura G, Motoyama T. Detection of HPV-DNA, *p53* alterations,

and methylation in penile squamous cell carcinoma in Japanese men. Pathol Int. 2008;58:477–82.

24. Lopes A, Bezerra AL, Pinto CA, Serrano SV, de Mello CA, Villa LL. p53 as a new prognostic factor for lymph node metastasis in penile carcinoma: analysis of 82 patients treated with amputation and bilateral lymphadenectomy. J Urol. 2002;168:81–6.

25. Campos RS, Lopes A, Guimarães GC, Carvalho AL, Soares FA. E-cadherin, MMP-2, and MMP-9 as prognostic markers in penile cancer: analysis of 125 patients. Urology. 2006;67:797–802.

26. Hegarty PK. MMP-2 and MMP-9 in lymph-node-positive bladder cancer. J Clin Pathol. 2012;65:470–1.

27. Gairdner D. The fate of the foreskin, a study of circumcision. BMJ. 1949;2:1433–7.

28. Oster J. Further fate of the foreskin. Incidence of preputial adhesions, phimosis, and smegma among Danish schoolboys. Arch Dis Child. 1968;43:200–3.

29. Morris BJ. Why circumcision is a biomedical imperative for the 21st century. Bioessays. 2007;29:1147–58.

30. Tseng HF, Morgenstern H, Mack T, et al. Risk factors for penile cancer: results of a population-based case–control study in Los Angeles County (United States). Cancer Causes Control. 2001;12:267–77.

31. Dillner J, von Krogh G, Horenblas S, et al. Etiology of squamous cell carcinoma of the penis. Scand J Urol Nephrol Suppl. 2000;205:189–93.

32. Nagpal BL, Prabhakar BR, Kataria SP, et al. Male genital tract tumors in Punjab, India. J Environ Pathol Toxicol Oncol. 1992;11:331–4.

33. Van Howe RS, Hodges FM. The carcinogenicity of smegma: debunking a myth. J Eur Acad Dermatol Venereol. 2006;20:1046–54.

34. O'Farrell N, Quigley M, Fox P. Association between the intact foreskin and inferior standards of male genital hygiene behaviour: a cross-sectional study. Int J STD AIDS. 2005;16:556–9.

35. Frisch M, Friis S, Kjaer SK, Melbye M. Falling incidence of penis cancer in an uncircumcised population (Denmark 1943–90). BMJ. 1995;311:1471.

36. Hegarty PK. Editorial on penile cancer: an analysis of socioeconomic factors at a southeastern tertiary referral center. Can J Urol. 2011;18:5528.

37. Zequi SD, Guimarães GC, da Fonseca FP, Ferreira U, de Matheus WE, Reis LO, et al. Sex with animals (SWA): behavioral characteristics and possible association with penile cancer. A multicenter study. J Sex Med. 2012;9(7):1860–7.

38. Tam DW, Van Scott EJ, Urbach F. Bowen's disease and squamous cell carcinoma. Occurrence in a patient with psoriasis after topical, systemic, and PUVA therapy. Arch Dermatol. 1979;115:203–4.

39. Stern RS. Genital tumors among men with psoriasis exposed to psoralens and ultraviolet A radiation (PUVA) and ultraviolet B radiation. The Photochemotherapy Follow-up Study. N Engl J Med. 1990;322:1093–7.

40. Stern RS. PUVA Follow-Up Study. The risk of squamous cell and basal cell cancer associated with psoralen and ultraviolet A therapy: a 30-year prospective study. J Am Acad Dermatol. 2012;66:553–62.

41. McIntyre M, Weiss A, Wahlquist A, Keane T, Clarke H, Savage S. Penile cancer: an analysis of socioeconomic factors at a southeastern tertiary referral center. Can J Urol. 2011;18:5524–8.

42. Harish K, Ravi R. The role of tobacco in penile carcinoma. BJU Int. 1995;75:375.

43. Minhas S, Manseck A, Watya S, Hegarty PK. Penile cancer—prevention and premalignant conditions. Urology. 2010;76:S24–35.

44. Giuliano AR. Human papillomavirus vaccination in males. Gynecol Oncol. 2007;107:S24–S6.

45. Elbasha EH, Dasbach EJ, Insinga RP. Model for assessing human papillomavirus vaccination strategies. Emerg Infect Dis. 2007;13:28–41.

46. Moses S, Bailey RC, Ronald AR. Male circumcision: assessment of health benefits and risks. Sex Transm Infect. 1998;74:368–73.

47. Circumcision policy statement.American Academy of Pediatrics Task Force on Circumcision, et al. Pediatrics. 2012;130(3):585–6.

48. Hutchinson J. On the influence of circumcision in preventing syphilis. Med Times Gazette. 1855;2:542–3.

49. Castellsague X, Bosch FX, Munoz N, Meijer CJ, Shah KV, de Sanjose S, et al. Male circumcision, penile human papillomavirus infection, and cervical cancer in female partners. N Engl J Med. 2002;346:1105–12.

50. Gray RH, Kigozi G, Serwadda D, Makumbi F, Watya S, Nalugoda F, et al. Male circumcision for HIV prevention in men in Rakai, Uganda: a randomised trial. Lancet. 2007;369:657.

51. Cathcart P. Trends in paediatric circumcision and its complications in England between 1997 and 2003. Br J Surg. 2006;93:885–90.

52. Wen LM, Estcourt CS, Simpson JM, et al. Risk factors for the acquisition of genital warts: are condoms protective? Sex Transm Infect. 1999;75:312–6.

53. Winer RL, Hughes JP, Feng Q, et al. Condom use and the risk of genital human papillomavirus infection in young women. N Engl J Med. 2006;354:2645–54.

54. Bleeker MC, Hogewoning CJ, Voorhorst FJ, et al. Condom use promotes regression of human papillomavirus-associated penile lesions in male sexual partners of women with cervical intraepithelial neoplasia. Int J Cancer. 2003;107:804–10.

55. Bleeker MC, Berkhof J, Hogewoning CJ, et al. HPV type concordance in sexual couples determines the effect of condoms on regression of flat penile lesions. Br J Cancer. 2005;92:1388–92.

Brant A. Inman, Suzanne B. Stewart,
and Michael W. Kattan

Abbreviations

AJCC	American Joint Committee on Cancer
CT	Computed tomography
CXR	Chest radiograph
DSNB	Dynamic sentinel lymph node biopsy
EAU	European Association of Urology
FDG-PET	^{18}F fluorodeoxyglucose positron emission tomography
GUONE	Gruppo Uro-Oncologico Del Nord Est
HPV	Human papillomavirus
LNMRI	Lymphotropic nanoparticle MRI
mm	Millimeters
MRI	Magnetic resonance imaging
PET	Positron emission tomography
SEER	Surveillance, Epidemiology, and End Results
TNM	Tumor, node and metastasis
US	Ultrasonography

B.A. Inman, M.D., M.S. (✉) • S.B. Stewart, M.D.
Division of Urology, Department of Surgery,
Duke University Medical Center,
Box 2812 DUMC, Durham, NC 27710, USA
e-mail: brant.inman@duke.edu

M.W. Kattan, Ph.D.
Department of Quantitative Health Sciences,
Cleveland Clinic, Cleveland, OH, USA

Staging Systems for Penile Cancer

For penile carcinoma many staging systems have been developed over time and are historically reflected in the literature [1, 2]. Accurate tumor staging is imperative in the management of the majority of malignancies and penile cancer is no exception. Staging provides a guide for the correct designation of therapeutic strategies and an indication of prognosis.

Jackson Staging System

The Jackson staging system was introduced in 1966 [2] and was the most commonly used staging classification for penile cancer up to the development of the tumor, node and metastasis (TNM) system created by the International Union Against Cancer and the American Joint Committee on Cancer. The Jackson classification (Table 2.1) stratifies penile cancer based on the operability of tumor and nodal metastases. Within this system, there is no description of the primary lesion such as the size or depth of invasion and no reference is made regarding its histological features.

TNM/AJCC Staging System

The TNM classification is the most widely recognized and currently used staging methodology for penile cancer (Tables 2.2, 2.3, 2.4, and 2.5).

Table 2.1 Jackson classification for penile carcinoma

Stage	Description
I	Confined to glans of prepuce
II	Invasion into shaft or corpora
III	Operable inguinal lymph node metastasis
IV	Tumor invades adjacent structures; inoperable inguinal lymph node metastasis

Table 2.2 2010 TNM staging of penile cancer—primary tumor (T) and histopathologic grading

T—primary tumor	
Tx	Primary tumor cannot be assessed
T0	No evidence of primary tumor
Tis	Carcinoma in situ
Ta	Noninvasive verrucous carcinoma, not associated with destructive invasion
T1	Tumor invades subepithelial connective tissue
T1a	Tumor invades subepithelial connective tissue without lymphovascular invasion and is not poorly differentiated or undifferentiated (T1 G1–2)
T1b	Tumor invades subepithelial connective tissues with lymphovascular invasion or is poorly differentiated or undifferentiated (T1 G3–4)
T2	Tumor invades corpus spongiosum/corpora cavernosa
T3	Tumor invades urethra
T4	Tumor invades other adjacent structures
G—histopathologic grade	
Gx	Grade of differentiation cannot be assessed
G1	Well differentiated
G2	Moderately differentiated
G3–4	Poorly differentiated/undifferentiated

Source: Edge SB, Byrd DR, Compton CC, Fritz AG, Greene FL, Trotti A, eds. AJCC Cancer Staging Handbook. 7th ed. New York: Springer; 2010

Table 2.3 2010 TNM staging of penile cancer—regional lymph nodes (N)

Clinical stage definition[a]	
cNx	Regional lymph nodes cannot be assessed
cN0	No palpable or visibly enlarged inguinal lymph node
cN1	Palpable mobile unilateral inguinal lymph node
cN2	Palpable mobile multiple or bilateral inguinal lymph nodes
cN3	Fixed inguinal nodal mass or pelvic lymphadenopathy, unilateral or bilateral
Pathologic stage definition[b]	
pNx	Regional lymph nodes cannot be assessed
pN0	No regional lymph node metastasis
pN1	Intranodal metastasis in a single inguinal lymph node
pN2	Metastasis in multiple or bilateral inguinal lymph nodes
pN3	Metastasis in pelvic lymph node(s), unilateral or bilateral or extranodal extension of regional lymph node metastasis

Source: Edge SB, Byrd DR, Compton CC, Fritz AG, Greene FL, Trotti A, eds. AJCC Cancer Staging Handbook. 7th ed. New York: Springer; 2010
[a]Clinical stage definition based on palpation and imaging
[b]Pathologic stage definition based on biopsy or surgical excision

Table 2.4 2010 TNM staging of penile cancer—distant metastasis (M)

M0	No distant metastasis
M1	Distant metastasis[a]

Source: Edge SB, Byrd DR, Compton CC, Fritz AG, Greene FL, Trotti A, eds. AJCC Cancer Staging Handbook. 7th ed. New York: Springer; 2010
[a]Lymph node metastasis outside of the true pelvis in addition to visceral or bone sites

Table 2.5 2010 TNM staging of penile cancer—anatomic stage

Stage 0	Tis	N0	M0
	Ta	N0	M0
Stage I	T1a	N0	M0
Stage II	T1b	N0	M0
	T2	N0	M0
	T3	N0	M0
Stage IIIa	T1–3	N1	M0
Stage IIIb	T1–3	N2	M0
Stage IV	T4	Any N	M0
	Any T	N3	M0
	Any T	Any N	M1

Source: Edge SB, Byrd DR, Compton CC, Fritz AG, Greene FL, Trotti A, eds. AJCC Cancer Staging Handbook. 7th ed. New York: Springer; 2010

The *T* stage is defined by the depth of tumor invasion, the *N* stage by the number and/or location of lymph nodes, and the *M* stage by the presence of distant metastases. The penile cancer TNM classification was first published in 1968 and has undergone multiple revisions with the latest update provided in 2010 [3]. This updated version includes subcategorization of T1 into T1a and T1b based on histopathological grading and lymphovascular invasion (Table 2.2). Both these histological elements have been found to be important in predicting lymph node metastases [4] and as a result the new subclassification of T1b is categorized as stage II, instead of its previous designation as stage I (Table 2.5). Additional changes to the 2010 TNM staging include prostate invasion being now classified as T4 as opposed to T3 and any lymph node involvement being considered as stage III or higher.

Even with the 2010 update, there continues to be debate regarding the appropriate TNM classification for penile cancer. One of these controversies involves the definition of T2. Currently, the T2 category contains primary tumors that involve either the corpus spongiosum and/or the corpora cavernosa. However, multiple studies have shown that tumor invasion into the cavernosa body represents an independent adverse prognostic factor for survival [5–7]. Specifically, Leijte et al. found that the 5-year disease specific survival for patients with corpora cavernosa invasion was significantly lower than that for patients with only corpus spongiosum invasion (52.6% versus 77.7%, respectively; $p=0.001$) [8]. There has also been question regarding the utility of the T3 category which defines tumor invading into the urethra. Arguments have been that superficial tumors located at the meatus can invade into the urethra, but not involve the spongiosum and/or cavernosal bodies. These tumors are often treated with only penile preserving methods which result in durable responses despite being classified as T3 [9]. Proposals to redefine T2 and T3 categories have been suggested but are not yet reflected in the current AJCC TNM classification for penile cancer.

Imaging Studies Useful for Staging Penile Cancer

Historically, imaging has not improved the accuracy of clinical staging. When clinical staging has been compared to pathologic findings, Horenblas et al. found that 26% of primary penile lesions and 20% of inguinal lymph nodes were staged incorrectly. Computed tomography (CT) and lymphography were not found to improve these results [10]. The available radiological modalities were not able to delineate anatomical tissue planes or to determine metastatic involvement of lymph nodes. However, with the advent of magnetic resonance imaging (MRI) and combined positron emission tomography (PET)-CT as well as lymphotropic nanoparticle enhanced MRI, the ability of radiology to enhance the precision of clinical staging using the TNM system is finally within reach.

Penile Imaging

Cavernosography

Corpus cavernosography has been used to detect both penile carcinoma as well as metastatic disease to the penis. The injection of contrast media directly into the corpora may show filling defects suggestive of tumor extension or metastatic seeding [11, 12]. Raghavaiah preformed cavernosography on ten patients preoperatively and found that this imaging modality successfully staged patients when compared with pathological exam. From clinical evaluation, cavernosogram upstaged one patient and two others were found to have tumor extension more proximally than was determined by palpation [13]. Cavernosography has also been used to identify nodular filling defects suggestive of metastases [14, 15].

Currently, cavernosography is not a modality that is commonly used in the evaluation of penile carcinoma. It is limited in its ability to evaluate tumor extension beyond the corporal bodies. Furthermore, noninvasive techniques, such as CT and MRI, have been developed which provide more comprehensive assessment of tumor involvement for both staging and surgical planning.

Sonography

Ultrasonography (US) is another imaging modality that has been investigated as an adjunct to clinical staging of penile carcinoma. In the majority of the literature, penile squamous cell carcinoma typically presents as a hypoechoic lesion with a heterogeneous appearance under ultrasound guidance [16–18]. However, variation in echogencity can be observed. Specifically, Agrawal et al. found that in 59 patients with penile carcinoma, 36% of the lesions were hyperechoic (21 cases), 47% were hypoechoic (28 cases), and 17% showed mixed echogenicity (10 cases). No significant association was found between echogenicity and tumor morphology or grade [16].

US has shown efficacy in differentiating tumor involvement among specific penile tissue planes. Clear relationships between tumor and the tunica albuginea, corpus cavernosum and spongiosum, and urethra have been documented using ultrasound [17, 18]. Delineation of tumor involvement with the glans penis proves however more difficult. Horenblas et al. found that US was not able to differentiate between invasion of tumor into the subepithelial tissue as opposed to the corpus spongiosum at the level of the glans [18]. Despite this limitation, US was found to enhance the accuracy of clinical staging for penile carcinoma overall by improving the estimation of local tumor extension. In the 2004 European Association of Urology (EAU) guidelines on penile cancer, US was proposed as the initial diagnostic modality of choice to assist the physical examination in assessing the depth of tumor invasion, particularly if corpora cavernosum infiltration is suspected [19].

Overall, the delineation of tissue structures with US suggests a clinical applicability for this imaging modality in the staging of penile carcinoma. The strengths of this technique compared to alternatives are its low cost and noninvasive nature. However, ultrasound is limited by its marked operator dependence and ability to clearly evaluate tumor extension beyond the base of penis [17, 20, 21]. Ultimately, the enhanced resolution capacity of CT and MRI has limited US widespread utilization.

Computed Tomography and Positron Emission Tomography

Historically, CT has been a modality with limited applicability due in large part by its poor soft tissue discrimination and imaging in only an uniplanar, axial format. Over time, through the development of helical scanning and multiplanar reconstruction, CT is now able to perform multidimensional imaging. However, it continues to have limited accuracy in contrast resolution of soft tissue planes. Therefore, CT has not become an imaging modality of choice for evaluating the primary lesion of penile cancer [11, 12].

There has been little published information on the use of PET/CT in the detection and "T" stage characterization of penile cancer. One study by Scher et al., found that in 13 patients with penile cancer, the pattern of fluorodeoxyglucose (FDG) uptake exhibited was typical of malignancy. Detection of the primary malignancy with PET/CT showed a sensitivity of 75% (6 of 8 lesions) and specificity of 75% (3 of 4 lesions). However, the ability of this combined imaging modality to accurately discern the extent of local invasion and ultimately the "T" stage remained limited due to its lack of soft tissue discrimination [22].

Magnetic Resonance Imaging

Currently, MRI represents the most sensitive imaging modality for the local staging of penile carcinoma. This technique has both superior soft tissue contrast and spatial resolution compared to alternative imaging studies such as US and CT. The addition of MRI provides enhanced anatomic detail for the evaluation of penile tumor extension indiscernible by physical examination. This anatomic detail allows for a more accurate designation of clinical "T" stage and precise surgical planning.

Penile carcinoma is preferentially evaluated on T2-weighted sequences on account of the superior contrast resolution between the hypointense tunica albuginea and hyperintense corporal bodies. Squamous cell carcinoma of the penis typically appears as a hypointense lesion compared to the adjacent corpora on both T1- and T2-weighted images [23–25]. With contrast enhanced imaging, these lesions show an increase in signal intensity but to a lesser degree than the normal corporal bodies [24]. Many studies concur that the value of contrast enhanced MRI for penile cancer is limited. Compared to T2-weighted images, use of gadolinium was not found to provide any additional information and was not helpful in determining primary tumor margins [26, 27].

Patient positioning is of vital importance to facilitate optimal soft tissue resolution during magnetic resonance imaging. Various techniques have been reported which include imaging the erect penis after intracavernosal injection of prostaglandin E1 as well as using endoluminal coils, such as endorectal or endovaginal coils during imaging. In the flaccid penis, conventional MRI has been reported to be limited in its ability to distinguish tumors confined to the tunica albuginea from those invading into the corporal bodies. At times, the corporal bodies may have a low T2 signal intensity due to fibrosis or a transiently reduced blood flow when the penis is flaccid.

This decreased signal intensity can cause the interface between the corporal bodies and the tunica albuginea, which naturally has a low T2 signal intensity, to be difficult to distinguish [26]. Imaging the erect penis holds the advantage of both increasing the image size and most importantly accentuating the boundary between the tunica albuginea and the corpora cavernosum on T2-weighted sequences. The increased blood flow resulting from the erection leads to a significantly stronger signal intensity of the corpora cavernosum and thereby greater contrast against the tunica albuginea [26–28].

Intercavernosal Alprostadil

Many reports have shown accurate local staging of penile cancer using MRI in conjunction with intracavernosal prostaglandin E1. In 2004, Scardino et al. found that MRI with erection correctly staged eight out of nine patients. The failure resulted from a lack of detection by MRI of a carcinoma in situ lesion. However, clinical examination did detect this lesion and allowed for appropriate treatment decisions to be carried out. In this series, two patients were upstaged after imaging, where MRI with erection detected involvement of the corpus spongiosum. As a result of these findings, the two patients underwent a partial penectomy, the appropriate surgical treatment for the designated stage tumor. This is in contrast to the initial treatment recommendation of laser resection that was based on the lower clinical stage as determined by physical exam [27]. This study was later confirmed by Petralia et al. who similarly found that MRI with erection provided correct staging in 12 out 13 patients with penile carcinoma. Clinical exam alone was found to only result in the correct staging of 8 out of 13 patients, with overstaging in two patients and understaging in three patients. Based on these findings, the authors concluded that MRI in conjunction with intracavernosal prostaglandin E1 augmented local staging capability of the physical exam and led to appropriate surgical planning [26].

In 2007, Kayes et al. confirmed the accurate staging capacity of MRI with intracavernosal prostaglandin E1 in a much larger cohort of 55 patients with penile carcinoma. The authors found that MRI precisely predicted corporal cavernosum involvement in all cases of pathologically confirmed disease. Stage-specific sensitivities and specificities of MRI with erection were determined to be as follows: T1 (85%, 83%), T2 (75%, 89%), and T3 (88%, 98%) [28]. Although this method of imaging has proven useful over clinical exam alone, MRI with erection has not been compared in the literature against the accuracy of staging by MRI without a pharmacologically induced penile erection. This comparison would be of utility as there are contraindications and cautions for the use of intracavernosal prostaglandin E1. Alprostadil, the commonly used intracavernosal prostaglandin E1 analog, is contraindicated in patients with penile implants and is cautioned for use in patients with anatomic abnormalities, such a tumors invading into the corporal bodies, as well as in patients with bleeding or coagulation disorders. As a result, some medical centers reserve the use of erection with MRI only when clinical uncertainty remains after imaging the flaccid penis [23, 25].

Endoluminal Coils

Alternatively to inducing an artificial erection, placement of endoluminal coils during MRI has also been shown to improve soft tissue resolution. Conventional imaging with MRI for penile and urethral carcinoma includes use of a surface or body coil typically placed over the pelvis. Endoluminal coil technology refers to the placement of a coil within a body cavity adjacent to the imaging tissue of interest. Endorectal, endovaginal, and endourethral coil MRI have all been investigated in imaging the pelvic floor and underlying penile/urethral pathology. Multiple reports have shown that using an endoluminal coil resulted in improved signal to noise ratio and higher tissue resolution [29, 30] as compared to conventional body coil MRI [31] as well as alternative imaging modalities [32]. In particular, these coils have allowed greater anatomic detail of ligamentous structures. To the authors' knowledge, endoluminal coil technology has not been specifically investigated in cases of penile carcinoma. However, it is likely that the benefits of

endoluminal coil MRI could be extrapolated to the majority of penile pathological processes. Unfortunately, one of the drawbacks of this technology is that it is not universally available nor routinely preformed. Furthermore, endoluminal probes can be uncomfortable for the patient and maybe not feasible in cases of an obstructing penile carcinoma.

Overall, MRI, even in its conventional form, signifies the most sensitive imaging modality for determining the local extension of penile and urethral carcinoma. The ability of MRI to augment physical examination and increase the accuracy of clinical staging leads to improved treatment planning. Ultimately, this enhanced staging capability and decision-making translates for the patient into better treatment outcomes and decreased morbidity.

Inguinal Imaging

One of the most important prognostic parameters for penile cancer is the presence and extent of lymph node involvement [33]. Physical exam is the initial method by which inguinal lymph node status is assessed [19]. The location of the primary lesion dictates the likely site of lymphatic spread. Penile tumors located at the prepuce and skin drain into the superficial inguinal nodes. Lymphatic vessels of the glans penis drain into the deep inguinal and external iliac nodes and that of the corporal bodies follows the internal iliac lymph nodes [23, 34]. The cross communication of this lymphatic system commonly results in bilateral lymph node disease even in the presence of unilateral penile tumors [19, 33].

In penile cancer, 30–60% of patients have palpable inguinal lymphadenopathy; however, nearly half of these detected nodes on exam are reactive [19, 33, 35]. Furthermore, up to 25% of patients with nonpalpable disease have been found to harbor occult inguinal metastases [5, 33, 36, 37]. Thus, based on these limitations of physical exam in detecting lymph node disease in penile carcinoma, the 2004 EUA guidelines have suggested that regional lymph nodes be evaluated weeks after treatment of the primary lesion.

Similarly, use of antibiotics has also been common practice to help distinguish inflammatory nodal reaction from metastatic disease [34, 38]. Lymph nodes that remain palpable following treatment of the primary penile lesion and/or after antibiotic therapy have a reported 90% likelihood of harboring a metastatic focus [38].

Radical lymph node dissection has been deemed as the most reliable staging method for lymph node involvement as well as constituting a potential curative intervention for nodal metastases. For penile cancer, it has been referred to as the "gold standard" for lymph node staging [36]. However, inguinal lymphadenectomy is associated with a high complication rates ranging from 30 to 50% and a mortality rate exceeding 1% [19, 33]. Common complications reported include severe lymphedema, skin flap necrosis, wound infection, and seroma formation [39]. Thus, subjecting all patients with penile cancer to a radical groin dissection would cause undue morbidity and overtreatment for many patients. Inguinal lymphadenectomy is strongly recommended in penile cancer with palpable nodal disease and positive histopathology [19]. However, the dilemma arises on how to proceed in cases of clinically negative lymph nodes and how to enhance accuracy of detecting true metastases in palpable lymph nodes at presentation in penile cancer. For these particular patients, a precise and less invasive method of lymph node staging is sought. Currently, there are a variety of imaging studies available which attempt to differentiate lymph node involvement morphologically or functionally.

Cross-sectional Imaging

US, CT, and MRI differentiate lymph node involvement through morphology. High resolution US evaluates lymph nodes based on size, shape, outline, and echogencity of its hilum. Subtle malignant changes in lymph node architecture are able to be detected via US and include asymmetric thickening and focal lobulations of the cortex in early disease and cortical thickening and loss of the hilum which is seen in advanced disease. Many of these changes evolve before the lymph node enlarges [35, 40]. Findings also suggestive of malignancy include loss of hilar sinus fat and progressive low echogenicity of the cortex. Color Doppler US can be useful in evaluating changes in the pattern of lymph node vascularity. In general, metastatic nodes have been found to display a peripheral vascularity whereas reactive nodes exhibit a hilar perfusion pattern [41]. In a recent report of 64 patients with clinically node negative squamous cell carcinoma of the penis, US was found to have a sensitivity and specificity of 74% and 77%, respectively, in the detection of occult inguinal metastases. As a result, the authors concluded that US alone was not an adequate staging method [42].

The technique of fine needle aspiration cytology was added to US studies in an effort to improve the diagnostic accuracy of identifying metastatic inguinal lymph nodes. In patients with squamous cell carcinoma of the vulva, this technique has yielded a sensitivity and specificity of 93% and 100%, respectively [43]. However, in penile cancer, the results have not been as robust. One study showed that in 83 clinically node negative inguinal regions, the combination of fine needle aspiration and US resulted in a sensitivity and specificity of 39% and 100%, respectively. Additionally, the majority of metastases that were detected occurred in nodes greater than 2 mm in size [44]. This demonstrates that US remains dependent on lymph node enlargement to identify metastases despite the addition of a host of cytological techniques.

CT and MRI are both similarly reliant on changes in lymph node size rather than architectural changes to determine the suspicion of metastasis. However, the use of size criteria to determine the presence of malignancy is nonspecific as lymph nodes in penile cancer frequently undergo reactive enlargement. As a result, cross sectional imaging can lead to a high false positive rate [45]. MRI does have the benefit of using differences in signal intensity to aid in detection. Even without nodal enlargement, if the signal intensity is similar to the primary tumor, then the lymph node should be considered suspicious of malignancy. Findings of central necrosis within lymph nodes also increase the likelihood of metastatic disease [33]. One advantage that both CT and MRI hold over US is that these modalities allow for the evaluation of occult metastases in the deep inguinal and pelvic nodes. Ultimately, all these cross sectional imaging studies are limited in their assessment for micrometastases.

PET/CT

PET/CT is a noninvasive imaging modality that allows for lymph node disease to be evaluated both functionally and morphologically. This technique has been assessed in both clinically node positive and node negative patients with penile cancer. Graafland et al. evaluated the ability of PET/CT to detect pelvic lymph node disease in 18 penile cancer patients with cytologically proven inguinal metastases. In such patients, PET/CT showed a sensitivity of 91%, a specificity of 100%, a positive predictive value of 100% and a negative predictive value of 94% in detecting pelvic nodal disease. Although this imaging modality revealed a high diagnostic accuracy, its restricted spatial resolution leads to inevitable false negative findings. Specifically, PET/CT remains limited in detecting microscopic nodal disease which are less than 2 mm in size [46]. The sensitivity of PET/CT in detecting positive lymph node disease has been found to increase with increasing nodal size [47] and tumor burden [48].

When PET/CT was evaluated for the detection of occult inguinal metastases in patients with penile cancer, the diagnostic accuracy was found to be poor. Leijte et al. found that in 24 patients with clinically node negative disease, PET/CT only correctly predicted one out of five tumor positive groins. All false negative findings occurred in lymph nodes of less than or equal to 10 mm. In contrast, PET/CT did have a specificity of 92% in this patient cohort, with 34 out of 37 negative groins correctly predicted [49]. This study showed that in patients with clinically negative nodes as determined by physical examination, PET/CT did not enhance the staging accuracy. For penile and urethral cancer, it is in

these patients with nonpalpable inguinal nodes that the evaluation of micrometastatic nodal disease is of vital importance. Unfortunately, current imaging tools remain limited in this realm.

Lymphotropic Nanoparticle Enhanced MRI

Lymphotropic nanoparticle enhanced MRI (LNMRI) is a promising noninvasive imaging modality recently introduced for lymph node staging in penile cancer. Lymphotropic nanoparticles are ultra-small coated particles of iron oxide, USPIOs, ferumoxtran-10 which are uniquely used as the contrast agent. The nanoparticles are captured by functioning macrophages present in normal lymph nodes. This results in a homogenous low signal on T2 weighted imaging. Nodes with metastatic disease either completely lack or have minimal normal phagocytes available to take up these nanoparticles. As a result, metastatic nodes show either absent or heterogenous signal intensity on MRI T2-weighted images [23, 34, 35].

Tabatabaei et al. examined this novel technique in seven patients with penile cancer, of which two had clinically palpable lymph node disease. Lymphotropic nanoparticle enhanced MRI results were compared to the histological examination of a total of 113 lymph nodes harvested during inguinal lymphadenectomy. This imaging modality was found to have a sensitivity of 100%, specificity of 97%, positive predictive value of 81%, and negative predictive value of 100%. The authors concluded that the low positive predictive value was secondary to nodal fibrosis mimicking small tumor deposits. They emphasized that the strong negative predictive value of this technique results in the low likelihood of missing patients who are in need of a therapeutic inguinal lymphadenectomy. This high accuracy of detecting negative disease may also allow for proceeding confidently with unilateral groin dissections as compared to the recommended bilateral lymphadenectomy when only unilateral inguinal lymphadenopathy is present. This imaging modality proved unique in that it was able to accurately diagnose metastatic disease in both patients with clinically positive and negative inguinal disease [50]. Although the results were impressive, as commented by Kroon et al., this technique is based on the scope of MRI at 1.5 T which is limited in spatial resolution for detecting metastases to approximately 1–2 mm [51]. This commentary hence called into question the ability of lymphotrophic nanoparticle enhanced MRI to detect micrometastatic disease.

In addition to being potentially limited by these features of MRI, lymphotrophic nanoparticle enhanced MRI is hindered by the time consuming and operator dependent interpretation of images. This technique requires radiologists to make node-by-node comparisons using the preliminary native MRI with the nanoparticle enhanced version. Based on the difficult methodology of interpretation and the limitation of micrometastases, Thoeny et al. investigated the combination of diffusion weighted MRI with nanoparticle technology in normal sized pelvic lymph nodes in 21 patients with bladder and prostate cancer. Diffusion weighted MRI provides structural information regarding the imaged tissue and allows uptake of nanoparticles within one exam thereby also providing cellular detail. The study showed that this modality correctly diagnosed 24 out of 26 positive nodes (92%) and was significantly shorter on average in the interpretation of radiological studies as compared to nanoparticle enhanced MRI (13 min versus 80 min). The two lymph nodes missed by the combination diffusion and nanoparticle technology were micrometastases which were less than 1 mm. Interestingly, this study used a 3 T MRI unit and continued to be limited in detecting micrometastases [52]. Thus, for both techniques of lymphotrophic nanoparticle and diffusion weighted MRI, further studies need to be performed in larger cohorts and with increasing MRI Tesla to determine the true potential of these modalities in overall staging efficacy and detecting micrometastases. Currently, nanoparticle technology is not routinely available; however, for penile and urethral cancer its future as a staging tool for lymph node disease appears promising.

Dynamic Sentinel Lymph Node Biopsy

Dynamic sentinel lymph node biopsy (DSNB) is a technique that uses a radiolabeled nanocolloid, technetium-99, to detect the location of sentinel nodes, which can then be removed and histologically examined for occult cancer cells. A sentinel node is theorized to be the first lymph node involved by metastasizing cancer cells from the primary tumor [23, 34]. DSNB is a well-established modality for lymph node evaluation in melanoma patients. In early stage melanoma, DSNB has resulted in a 5% false negative rate, a 10% complication rate, and a better disease-free survival for those patients who subsequently underwent a lymphadenectomy as a result of a positive DSNB as compared to patients undergoing observation [53]. DSNB has recently been investigated for the detection of occult lymph node disease in penile cancer.

The technique involves peritumoral intradermal injection of the radioisotope the day prior to surgery. After injection, lymphoscintigraphy is preformed in which images of the pelvis using a gamma camera are obtained. These images show the general anatomic location of the sentinel node allowing the overlying skin to be marked designating the site of the node(s). At surgery, blue dye is injected intradermally adjacent to the tumor allowing the lymph nodes draining the tumor to be visually identified. The sentinel node(s) are detected both visually by the blue coloration and the radioactivity through the use of a gamma probe. The node(s) with maximum radioactivity are then removed and examined histologically [23, 34].

In penile cancer, currently DSNB shows promise in the challenging area of detecting occult metastatic lymph node disease. Initially, DSNB was plagued by high false negative rates ranging from 22 to 75% [54–56]. The high false negative rate was initially attributed to suboptimal technique [54, 57, 58]. After instituting modifications, the false negative rate drastically decreased and DSNB became considered a potential lymph node staging modality for penile cancer [59]. Recent reports have demonstrated its improved efficacy. A prospective study performed in 2009 on 64 patients with clinical node negative penile cancer revealed that the combination of DSNB and US with or without fine needle aspiration cytology accurately identified occult nodal metastases. The authors felt that US alone was insufficient as a staging modality; however, the combination modality was favored for detecting occult nodal disease [42]. Leijte et al. confirmed the utility of DSNB in staging clinically node negative penile cancer in 323 patients treated across two separate centers. DSNB was found to have a sentinel node identification rate of 97%, a false negative rate of 7%, an overall complication rate of 4.7%, and virtually no learning curve required for the procedure [60]. Although invasive compared to alternative imaging modalities, DSNB appears efficacious and minimal risk in identifying occult metastatic disease in the clinical dilemma of a patient with clinically node negative penile cancer and high-risk features for occult nodal metastases.

Systemic Imaging

In penile cancer, distant metastases found at the time of clinical presentation are uncommon. Approximately 1.2–5% of patients with penile carcinoma have distant metastases. Lung, liver, and bone are the most common sites for hematogenous dissemination. The pubic bone, abdominal wall or scrotum can also be involved secondary to direct tumor extension. Typically, metastases to these sites occur with advanced stage and late in the course of disease. For patients with high stage disease, historic evaluation of distant metastases include a standard chest radiograph, radionuclide bone scan, and a CT of the abdomen and pelvis [11, 23, 38, 61]. The poor resolution of CT in detecting distant tumor spread has lead to the investigation of alternative modalities.

In the field of head and neck cancers, ^{18}F-labelled fluorodeoxyglucose (FDG)-PET scans have shown promise in detecting distant metastases effectively. FDG is a glucose analog that is taken up by metabolically active cells using glucose. As cancer cells typically have a higher metabolic rate than normal cells, FDG preferentially accumulates in malignancies [62].

Krabbe et al. recently found that whole body FDG-PET was superior to chest CT and chest radiograph (CXR) for staging of lung metastases in 149 patients with primary head and neck squamous cell carcinoma. Specifically, FDG-PET had a sensitivity and specificity of 92% and 93%, respectively; whereas, the sensitivity and specificity of chest CT was 74% and 61%, respectively and CXR was 41% and 91%, respectively. Based on these results, the authors proposed that FDG-PET should be considered as the initial staging modality for assessing the distant metastatic status [63].

PET in combination with CT has shown some efficacy in detecting distant metastatic disease among head and neck cancer patients. Gourin et al. found that PET/CT had a sensitivity and specificity of 86% and 84%, respectively, with a positive predictive value of 60% and negative predictive value of 95% in detecting both pulmonary and nonpulmonary metastatic sites among 64 patients with recurrent disease. The authors concluded that PET/CT should be performed in patients with suspected recurrent disease as part of their routine assessment [64].

The success of PET and PET/CT in the evaluation of distant metastatic disease among head and neck cancers can likely be extrapolated to penile cancer. However, there is a paucity of literature investigating the utility of PET/CT for this cancer type. One study has shown that PET/CT was effective in detecting distant metastases in penile cancer patients. PET/CT detected distant metastases in five patients of which four were confirmed histologically [46]. These results forecast a promising future for PET/CT in penile cancer. With corroborative studies on PET/CT in detecting distant metastatic disease for penile cancer, the historic modalities of CXR, bone scan, and CT will likely be replaced by this novel whole body imaging modality.

Penile Cancer Prognosis

Patient prognosis is one of the most important factors considered in medical decision-making. Physicians commonly tailor treatment recommendations based on expected survival and, similarly, patients alter their willingness to accept treatment-associated risk when faced with different prognoses. Many difficulties exist for the physician tasked with discussing prognostic information with a cancer patient including how much data to provide, how to be sensitive but honest when relaying bad news, and how to deal with specific individual, cultural and legal expectations [65]. While very little is known about the specific preferences and needs of men facing a diagnosis of penile cancer [66], research in other cancer populations has shown several important things:

- Most cancer patients want to be given prognostic information and consider it very important [65, 67].
- Most cancer patients want to know about the extent of spread, the probability of cure, and the side-effects of treatment [67, 68].
- Approximately 80% of patients want a qualitative prognosis (i.e., good, bad, long, short) and 50% want a quantitative prognosis (i.e., numerical expected survival estimate) [68].

There is therefore a good rationale for trying to arrive at accurate estimates of patient outcome. While prognosis should ideally include both the course (e.g., expected side-effects of therapy and complications of disease-progression) and outcome (e.g., expected duration of survival and probability of cure) of a particular disease, in this section survival is the primary prognostic outcome we consider.

Population Survival Estimates

The most basic prognosis that can be provided to a penile cancer patient is an unadjusted estimate of their expected survival, that is to say, an estimate that does not consider the specific characteristics of their cancer (e.g., stage, grade, etc.…) or their underlying health (e.g., age, comorbidity, etc.…). There are several different ways of calculating such an estimate and these are discussed individually below. However, prior to addressing these different methods of measuring survival, a brief comment is needed regarding data sources for survival estimation.

Penile cancer survival data are obtainable from three different sources: population-based cancer registries (e.g., SEER), institutional or individual case series (e.g., University Departments), and clinical trials (e.g., SWOG 8520). In general, survival estimates attained from population-based datasets are preferred wherever possible since they are subject to fewer selection biases than case-series or clinical trials [69–72]. This means that population-based studies are typically more generalizable [73], and for this reason we reference them herein whenever possible. However, population-based cancer registries have their own problems and inherent biases [74], and often lack the granular data needed for detailed prognostic tool construction.

It is also important not to confuse cancer mortality with cancer survival. Mortality rates refer to the overall mortality burden of a cancer in a population. For example, prostate cancer has double the mortality rate (24 deaths per 100,000 men at risk) of pancreatic cancer (12 deaths per 100,000 men at risk) in American men but has a 20-fold higher survival rate (>95% 5 year relative survival versus 6% relative survival) [75]. This is because prostate cancer is far more common than pancreatic cancer and mortality rates are metrics that are influenced by the cancer incidence rate whereas survival rates are not.

Survival Probability

The *survival probability* is the proportion of patients with a particular disease that do not die within a specified period of time [76]. By convention, the survival probability of most cancers is calculated over the 5-year time interval following diagnosis. Since survival data are positively skewed (i.e., the distribution of survival times has a longer right tail than left tail) and are subject to censoring (i.e., death has not been observed at the time of study closure), special analytic methods are required to estimate the survival probability. Three commonly used methods of estimating the survival probability are the actuarial life-table method, the Kaplan-Meier method, and the Nelson-Aalen method [77].

In oncology, the survival probability is often reported in two different forms: the overall survival probability and the cancer-specific survival probability (a.k.a. disease-specific survival, cause-specific survival). In the *overall survival probability* estimate, all deaths are counted toward the endpoint regardless of whether they were related to the underlying cancer or not [78]. The *cancer-specific survival probability* estimate only counts deaths that were directly or indirectly related to the cancer and censors patients that die from other competing causes as if they were lost to follow-up. Calculating cancer-specific survival requires accurate information on the cause of death, which is often missing in large datasets and is one reason why overall survival estimates are more commonly reported. Additionally, it can sometimes be difficult to determine whether a death was cancer-related or not [79]. For example, if a patient has a pulmonary embolism 2 weeks after inguinal lymphadenectomy, did they die from penile cancer? What if the embolism happened 2 months postoperatively? If a substantial amount of competing non-cancer deaths occur in the oncologic population of interest, the cancer-specific survival estimate may be somewhat biased [80]. In this circumstance, statistical methods that better address *competing mortality risks* may be preferred [81].

Population-level data from the Surveillance, Epidemiology, and End Results (SEER) program for penile cancer show an overall survival probability of 55% and a cancer-specific survival probability of 82% at 5 years [82]. However, the survival of penile cancer patients depends highly on certain prognostic factors and these estimates should be used only as a broad guide to prognosis.

Relative Survival

Another common way to express survival outcomes for population-level data is a measure called *relative survival*. The idea behind relative survival is simple: take the observed survival of cancer patients and divide it by their expected survival without necessarily having cancer to arrive at a ratio of observed/expected survival. The expected survival denominator is calculated from life tables from age, gender, and calendar year matched members of the general population. Race or ethnicity matching are also performed on occasion. Appropriate calculation of the expected survival estimates is very important and can be difficult in countries where accurate national vital statistics are not easily available. The beauty of the relative survival method is that cause of death information is not required since mortality from competing causes is accounted for in the expected survival denominator because the general population is subject to death from all causes. For population-level cancer registries, this is a big advantage since the precise cause of death in a cancer patient may be difficult to ascertain or assign [83].

Technically, there a few different ways of actually performing relative survival analysis and they differ mainly in the way that the expected survival denominator is calculated. The first method to become popular was suggested by Ederer in 1961 and has become known as the *Ederer I method* [84]. The Ederer I method doesn't account for censoring and therefore usually overestimates the relative survival ratio. The alternative *Ederer II method* does account for censoring but is dependent on the observed mortality and therefore usually underestimates the relative survival ratio [85]. Lastly, the *Hakulinen method* accounts for censoring but does not depend on the observed mortality and therefore tends to be the least biased method of calculating relative survival [86]. From a practical standpoint, the various relative survival estimates are not usually dramatically different from one another when looking at the 5-year endpoint. However, when assessing 10 or 15 year relative survival, more modern statistical innovations have allowed for relative survival regression [87].

Table 2.6 summarizes 5-year relative survival estimates for penile cancer obtained from several population-based cancer registries [88–94]. Despite being calculated in different populations and at different time periods, the overall 5-year relative survival estimates seem to converge at around 70% for penile cancer.

Case Fatality Ratio

A much less commonly used measure of cancer survival is the *case-fatality ratio*. The case-fatality ratio is the proportion of patients that have the disease of interest (i.e., penile cancer) that will ultimately die from it. The main problem with

Table 2.6 Population-based estimates of overall relative survival for penile cancer

Source	Years	References	Sample size	5-year relative survival (%)
USA (SEER[a])	1990–1994	[88, 89]	1,554	73
	2000–2004	[88, 89]	1,554	67
Denmark	2006–2010	[90, 94]	581	75
Norway	2005–2009	[90, 94]	426	80
Sweden	2005–2009	[90, 94]	908	69
Finland	2006–2010	[90, 94]	286	59
The Netherlands	1989–2006	[91]	1,883	79
UK	2001–2003	[92]	N/A	72
Europe (EUNICE[b])	1990–1994	[88, 89]	2,464	65
	2000–2004	[88, 89]	2,464	66
Europe (RARECARE[c])	2000–2002	[93]	1,555	69

[a]Surveillance, epidemiology, and end results program
[b]European network for indicators on cancer
[c]Surveillance of rare cancers in Europe

calculating traditional case-fatality ratios in chronic illnesses (like cancer) is that you have to follow patients until resolution of disease or death since censoring is not accounted for. For acute illnesses, like a viral outbreak, this is not a problem since the disease either kills or resolves within weeks to months. For cancer, however, years to decades may go by before the final outcome of a patient is known making calculation of the case-fatality ratio impractical. Newer methods of calculating the case-fatality ratio that account for censoring have been developed and may be more applicable to cancer patients [95].

Case fatality estimates for penile cancer are difficult to find, particularly for population-based datasets, which is likely a reflection of the problems of calculating this measure for cancer. One case-series from Jamaica reported a 38% case-fatality ratio but is unlikely representative of the larger population of penile cancer patients [96].

Patient-Related Prognostic Factors

The outcomes of patients depend not only on their diagnosis of penile cancer, but also on their overall state of health. Relatively little attention has been given to the impact of patient-related prognostic factors in penile cancer.

Age

Age is a key determinant of outcome for most diseases, including many cancers [97]. Older patients tend to have higher comorbidity burdens [98–100], different health preferences, and risk acceptance than younger patients [101]. In addition, older patients have an altered chemotherapy drug metabolism [102, 103], as well they may be perceived/treated differently by their physicians [104], and in some instances, have biologically distinct tumor characteristics [105, 106]. In the specific case of penile cancer, increasing age is associated with decreasing 5-year relative survival rates (Table 2.7) [88–90, 93, 107].

Multimorbidity

Multimorbidity is defined as the presence of several chronic conditions in an individual patient for a long period of time [100]. Multimorbidity is a slightly different concept than comorbidity since the underlying idea is that the net health effect of the summation of individual comorbidities (i.e., multiple morbidities) is greater than its constituent parts. The prevalence of multimorbidity increases strongly with age [99], and coincides with the age-dependent rise in incidence of penile cancer [91, 107, 109, 110]. Multimorbidity has been shown to increase overall and cancer-specific mortality rates in older men [111]. It therefore stands to reason that multimorbidity

Table 2.7 Age-stratified relative survival of men with penile cancer

Source	Years	References	Sample size	Age stratum	5-year relative survival (%)
USA (SEER[a])	1998–2003	[107]	131	<50	86[b]
			186	50–59	82[b]
			292	60–69	80[b]
			314	70–79	80[b]
			334	≥80	66[b]
USA (SEER)	2000–2004	[88, 89]	1,554	15–54	67
				55–64	72
				65–74	69
				≥75	62
Europe (EUNICE[c])	2000–2004	[88, 89]	2,464	15–54	73
				55–64	71
				65–74	61
				≥75	57
Europe (RARECARE[d])	2000–2002	[93]	681	<65	73
			888	>65	65
Denmark	2006–2010	[90]	581	<50	73
				50–59	84
				60–69	73
				70–79	76
				80–90	67
Norway	2005–2009	[90]	426	<50	71
				50–59	81
				60–69	79
				70–79	92
				80–90	65
Sweden	2005–2009	[90]	908	<50	81
				50–59	71
				60–69	69
				70–79	61
				80–90	73
Finland	2006–2010	[90]	286	<50	72
				50–59	78
				60–69	79
				70–79	44
				80–90	20

[a]Surveillance, epidemiology, and end results program
[b]Estimated from mortality/incidence ratios using the method of Asadzadeh Vostakolaei [108]
[c]European network for indicators on cancer
[d]Surveillance of rare cancers in Europe

patients with penile cancer are likely at higher risk of death than those without comorbidities. Currently, there are no published data on the prognostic implications of multimorbidity for penile cancer.

Tumor-Related Prognostic Factors

Tumor staging and pathological features identified within the tumor specimen are critical for establishing an accurate disease prognosis. Below are

Table 2.8 Relationship between local tumor stage (T) and regional (N) or systemic (M) metastases (SEER database 1973–2009) [114]

	Sample size	Ta (%)	Tis (%)	T1 (%)	T2 (%)	T3 (%)	T4 (%)
N stage							
N0	1,318	0.2[a]	0	69	19	11	1
N1	89	0	0	28	43	25	4
N2	91	0	0	37	27	27	8
N3	71	0	0	28	35	31	6
M stage							
M0	1,548	0.2	0	64	21	13	2
M1	48	0	0	35	25	31	8

[a]Row-wise percentages

several of the more important tumor-related prognostic factors for penile cancer.

Degree of Local Invasion (T Stage)

Disease stage is the most important prognostic factor of penile cancer outcome and the TNM staging system for penile cancer is described in detail in Sect. "Penile Imaging". The T stage is a measure of the local invasiveness of a penile tumor and is a key determining factor of disease outcome. The rate of lymph node and distant organ metastases increases dramatically with local tumor stage which is likely a key reason why tumor stage predicts survival (Table 2.7) [112]. The influence of disease stage on survival is shown in Table 2.8 [91, 113].

Tumor Depth (Thickness)

A precise method of quantifying the amount of cutaneous invasion by a tumor is to measure its depth of penetration or its thickness. Breslow first described the depth of tumor invasion as prognostic in melanoma in 1970 and separated the depth into five categories: <0.75 mm, 0.75–1.5 mm, 1.5–2.25 mm, 2.25–3.0 mm, and >3 mm [115]. Currently, the TNM system for melanoma has simplified the tumor depth into four categories: <1 mm, 1–2 mm, 2–4 mm and >4 mm, with each category demonstrating a significant impact on survival [116]. A closely related measure to the Breslow depth is the Clark level, which describes the anatomic level invasion of the skin [117]. Five Clark levels are defined: epidermis, papillary dermis, papillary and reticular dermis,

reticular dermis, and subcutaneous fat. Most studies find the Breslow depth superior to the Clark level for prognostic purposes. Since penile cancer is essentially a skin cancer of the penis, several groups have assessed metrics similar to the Breslow and Clark systems for their prognostic ability (Table 2.9). In general, the deeper the penile cancer is growing into the penis, the higher the likelihood of inguinal metastases and the worse the survival [4, 118–120]. A 5 mm or greater depth of invasion appears to impart a poor prognosis [53].

Lymph Node Metastasis (N Stage)

The inguinal lymph nodes are felt to be the first relay in the metastasis pathway of penile cancer, and therefore, the correct clinical staging of the inguinal lymph nodes is of paramount importance to disease outcome prognostication. A full discussion of the prognostic role of the inguinal lymph nodes is presented in Chap. 6. Here, we present population-based and select large case series survival outcomes of penile cancer patients stratified by lymph node status (Table 2.10). It is obvious from this table that survival drops precipitously with worsening lymph node involvement by cancer. More recently, extranodal extension of cancer has been shown to be associated with worse survival and for this reason such cases are considered to be in the N3 category [123, 124]. Similarly, a lymph node density (positive nodes/total nodes) above 5–10% predicts poor survival [125]. Resecting cancer-laden lymph nodes early on in the disease course is

Table 2.9 Relative survival of men with penile cancer stratified by tumor stage

Source	Years	References	Sample size	Stage group	Relative survival (%)
USA (SEER[a])	1973–2009	[114]	23	Ta	94[b]
			835	Tis	96[b]
			795	T1	73[b]
			269	T2	60[b]
			164	T3	62[b]
			31	T4	45[b]
The Netherlands	1989–2006	[91]	353	Stage 0	93[c]
			725	Stage I	89[c]
			329	Stage II	81[c]
			166	Stage III	50[c]
			62	Stage IV	20[d]

[a]Surveillance, epidemiology, and end results program
[b]5-year relative survival
[c]10-year relative survival
[d]2-year relative survival

Table 2.10 Inguinal lymph node positivity and tumor depth

Source	Years	References	Sample size	Tumor depth (mm)	Positive inguinal lymph nodes (%)
Italy (GUONE[a])	1980–2002	[119]	62	≤5	22
			91	>5	51
Brazil	1953–1985	[121]	39	≤5	33
			97	>5	58
Brazil	1996–2007	[122]	35	≤5	17
			161	>5	40
USA	1980–1997	[4]	22	≤5	36
			26	>5	38

[a]Gruppo Uro-Oncologico del Nord Est

therefore beneficial. In fact, several groups have shown that delaying lymphadenectomy results in worse survival outcomes [5, 37, 126, 127].

Lymphovascular Invasion

Lymphovascular invasion is defined as the invasion of endothelial-lined spaces located within or near the tumor by cancer cells and is a hallmark of cancer metastasis [131]. In the case of penile cancer where metastasis normally proceeds in an orderly fashion from the penis to the inguinal lymph nodes and then to the pelvic lymph nodes and beyond, lymphovascular invasion is probably the principal method of disease spread [132]. Lymphovascular invasion in penile cancer is associated with higher rates of inguinal lymph

node metastasis and decreased survival (Table 2.11) [4, 120, 122]. The probability of having lymphovascular invasion depends on the histologic subtype [133].

Perineural Invasion

Perineural invasion is the neoplastic invasion of nerves and it is another route of spread for tumors. Certain malignancies (e.g., head and neck cancers) appear to have a particular predilection for perineural spread and when identified in a pathology specimen, perineural invasion is usually an indicator of poor prognosis [135]. Penile cancer is not exception and several studies have shown increased inguinal lymph node metastasis rates and decreased survival in patients with tumors

Table 2.11 Survival of men with penile cancer stratified by inguinal lymph node status

Source	Years	References	Sample size	Lymph node status	Survival (%)
USA (SEER)	1973–2009	[114]	1,872	N0	85[a]
			80	N1	61[a]
			75	N2	34[a]
			58	N3	21[a]
			108	Nx	44[a]
The Netherlands	1989–2006	[91]	915	N0	90[b]
			247	N+	38[b]
			368	Nx	82[b]
USA (MDACC[c])	1956–2001		17	N1	81[d]
			4	N2	50[d]
			24	N3	41[d]
France	1986–2006	[128]	52	N0	93[d]
			29	N1	89[d]
			23	N2	31[d]
			10	N3	0[d]
India	1987–1998	[124]	26	N0	96[e]
			65	N1/2	65[e]
			54	N3	9[e]
Peru	1953–2001	[129]	87	N0	92[e]
			–	N1	100[e]
			–	N2	68[e]
			–	N3	31[e]
Italy (GUONE)	1980–2002	[130]	–	N0	94[d]
			–	N1	89[d]
			–	N2	7[d]
			–	N3	0[d]

[a]5-year relative survival
[b]10-year relative survival
[c]MD Anderson Cancer Center
[d]5-year cancer-specific survival
[e]5-year overall survival

demonstrating perineural invasion (Table 2.12) [120, 134, 136]. The probability of having perineural invasion also depends on the histologic subtype [133].

Distant Organ Metastases (M Stage)

The most dire prognostic feature in penile cancer is the presence of systemic metastases, a finding that is thought to be universally fatal. Most series combine metastatic cases with locally advanced cases (bulky inguinal, pelvic nodes, or T4 tumors) making the data extraction for metastatic patients difficult and often overestimated. The median survival of patients with metastatic penile cancer is approximately 8 months (Table 2.13).

Tumor Grade

Tumor grade is a critical prognostic factor for most human cancers and the first grading system of any cancer was described for squamous cell carcinomas of the lip [141]. The original Broders grading system had four grade categories (Grade 1 = well differentiated, Grade 2 = moderately differentiated, Grade 3 = poorly differentiated, Grade 4 = undifferentiated) but many contemporary pathologists lump grades 3 and 4 together [142]. While it is well established that tumor grading lacks reproducibility, it is still a very important prognostic factor and is closely related to tumor stage. For example, high grade tumors are more likely to have an advanced T stage,

Table 2.12 Inguinal lymph node positivity and lymphovascular invasion

Source	Years	References	Sample size	Lymphovascular invasion	Positive inguinal lymph nodes (%)
Italy (GUONE[a])	1980–2002	[119]	19	Absent	5
			7	Present	71
Paraguay	–	[134]	98	Absent	45
			36	Present	61
Canada	1997–2009	[120]	31	Absent	26 (50% dead)[b]
			12	Present	50 (83% dead)[b]
Brazil	1996–2007	[122]	157	Absent	29
			39	Present	64
Brazil	1953–1985	[121]	49	Absent	31
			85	Present	64
USA	1980–1997	[4]	27	Absent	11
			21	Present	71

[a]Gruppo Uro-Oncologico del Nord Est
[b]Mean follow-up 3.9 years

Table 2.13 Inguinal lymph node positivity and perineural invasion

Source	Years	References	Sample size	Perineural invasion	Positive inguinal lymph nodes (%)
Paraguay	–	[134]	86	Absent	38
			48	Present	69
Canada	1997–2009	[120]	34	Absent	29 (50% dead)[a]
			9	Present	44 (100% dead)[a]
Brazil	1996–2007	[122]	152	Absent	31
			44	Present	52

[a]Mean follow-up 3.9 years

Table 2.14 Relative survival of men with metastatic penile cancer

Source	Years	References	Sample size	5-year survival[a] (%)	Median survival (weeks)
USA (SEER[b])	1973–2009	[114]	39	8	34
The Netherlands Cancer Institute	1956–2006	[137]	10	0	20
The Netherlands Cancer Registry	1989–2006	[91]	16	20[c]	–
SWOG 8520	1986–1994	[138]	40	–	28
Italy	2004–2011	[139]	25	0	32
UK	1997–1999	[140]	9	0	–

[a]Cancer-specific survival
[b]Surveillance, epidemiology, and end results program
[c]2-year relative survival

more likely to be associated with lymph node metastases, and more likely to metastasize (Table 2.14) [142]. Consequently, increasing tumor grade is accompanied by a reduced patient survival as reported in most studies on penile cancer (Table 2.15).

Table 2.15 Stage-grade relationships in penile cancer (SEER database 1973–2009) [114]

	Sample size	Grade 1 (%)	Grade 2 (%)	Grade 3 (%)	Grade 4 (%)
T stage					
T1	785	39[a]	43	18	0.5
T2	315	23	48	26	2
T3	202	18	49	31	2
T4	22	18	50	32	0
N stage					
N0	1,047	37	44	18	0.5
N1	84	12	44	39	5
N2	80	13	50	36	1
N3	63	10	44	44	2
M stage					
M0	1,257	33	45	22	1
M1	41	12	34	49	5

[a]Row-wise percentages

Tumor Location on Penis

Penile cancers can be located on the glans penis (58%), prepuce (29%), shaft (7%) or in a combination of regions (6%) [144]. A recent analysis of SEER data suggests that the anatomic location of the tumor may affect prognosis [144]. Five-year relative survival was estimated at 83% for preputial tumors, 74% for glans tumors, 77% for shaft tumors, and 63% for tumors involving more than one anatomic zone.

Histologic Subtype

The histologic subtype of penile cancer has long been known to be of prognostic importance. For example, it has been known for nearly 90 years that verrucous carcinomas of the genitalia, even when very large in size, rarely metastasize [145]. The World Health Organization has developed consensus pathological criteria that allow penile skin tumors to be subcategorized into highly specific diagnostic bins [146]. For the squamous cell carcinomas that represent the vast majority of penile cancers, several subtypes have been identified and outcomes appear to vary according to subtype (Table 2.16).

Human Papilloma Virus

Squamous cell carcinomas are very frequently caused by human papilloma virus (HPV) infection and penile cancer is no exception [163]. While historical estimates of HPV positivity in penile cancer vary widely [164], modern reports using more sophisticated methods have shown that up to 85% of penile cancers have detectable HPV DNA [165]. The presence of HPV is not only important from a mechanistic standpoint but may also have prognostic and therapeutic relevance.

The best example of the prognostic importance of HPV is found in head and neck cancers, where approximately 25–50% of tumors are thought to be HPV-related [166–168]. HPV-positive head and neck tumors have been consistently shown to have a more favorable prognosis than HPV-negative tumors [166, 169, 170]. Additionally, the specific HPV genotype may also have prognostic relevance and do certain cell cycle markers (e.g., P16INK4a) which are associated with HPV infection [171–173].

In penile cancer, the prognostic role of HPV infection is less well established. For example, several groups have found no association between penile cancer HPV status and stage, grade, or lymph node positivity [165, 174, 175]. Contrarily, other groups have found HPV positive tumors to be of higher grade (implying potentially a worse prognosis) [176, 177]. And yet another group has found that HPV-positive penile cancers do better, akin to head and neck cancers [178]. These contrasting reports show the unclear relationship between HPV and penile cancer.

Table 2.16 Relative survival of men with penile cancer stratified by tumor grade

Source	Years	References	Sample size	Grade category	Relative survival (%)
USA (SEER[a])	1973–2009	[114]	1,122	Grade 1	85[b]
			1,417	Grade 2	64[b]
			654	Grade 3	54[b]
			47	Grade 4	54[b]
			3,684	Unknown	91[b]
The Netherlands	1989–2006	[91]	445	Grade 1	77[c]
			530	Grade 2	73[c]
			195	Grade 3	66[c]
India	1984–1987	[143]	66	Grade 1	90[d]
			64	Grade 2	59[d]
			12	Grade 3	17[d]

[a]Surveillance, epidemiology, and end results program
[b]5-year relative survival
[c]10-year relative survival
[d]5-year cancer-specific survival

Pathologic studies have demonstrated an association between HPV status and the development of specific penile cancer histologic subtypes, with basaloid and warty carcinomas being most frequently associated with HPV [179, 180]. Different molecular pathways appear to be activated in HPV-positive and negative penile cancers implying that optimization of targeted therapy for penile cancers may require knowledge of the patient's HPV status [181, 182]. Lastly, though HPV vaccination has been clearly shown to reduce the incidence of HPV-associated genital lesions in males (i.e., condylomata, intraepithelial neoplasia, and cancers) [183], it is unknown whether HPV vaccination could help men with established penile cancer.

Molecular Markers

Many molecular markers have been tested for their prognostic ability in penile cancer. Table 2.17 summarizes key results of interest.

Gene expression profiling has also been done in a limited number of patients with penile cancer. Kroon et al. constructed a 44-probe classifier in 70 patients with penile cancer but the classifier was not found to be clinically useful [194].

Comprehensive Prognostic Tools in Penile Cancer

Above is a description of individual prognostic factors that are important and relevant in penile cancer. While knowing these individual factors can certainly help with prognostication at the patient level, it is better to consider combinations of these variables to arrive at more precise estimates of patient outcome. Prognostic tools (i.e., nomograms, risk groupings, risk scores, etc....) attempt to combine several variables into one meaningful model that predicts disease outcome. In the case of penile cancer, there are a few such tools and we review these here.

Solsona and European Association of Urology (EAU) Risk Groups

One of the earliest and simplest prognostic tools for penile cancer was proposed by Solsona [6]. Based on tumor stage and grade as well as data from a small series of 66 patients, he proposed three simple risk categories for penile cancer (Table 2.18). Low risk patients had a 0% probability of inguinal lymph node metastases,

Table 2.17 Penile cancer histologic subtype and outcome

Subtype	References	Sample size	Lymph node metastases (%)	Dead of cancer (%)	5-year relative survival (%)
Squamous cell carcinomas	[114]	6,401	–	–	81
Usual/conventional	[133]	215	28	20	
Mixed	[133]	32	9	3	
Verrucous	[133]	24	0	0	
Warty	[133]	23	17	9	
Papillary	[133]	17	12	6	
Basaloid	[133]	14	50	21	
	[147]	20	71	50	
Sarcomatoid	[133]	4	75	75	
	[148]	15	89	–	
	[149]	12	50	67	
Adenosquamous	[133]	4	50	0	
Basal cell carcinoma	[114]	50	–	–	85
Sarcomas					
Kaposi's sarcoma	[150]	21	–	0[a]	
	[151]	189	–	11[a]	
Leiomyosarcoma	[152]	14	7	–	
	[153]	29	–	28	
	[114]	16			64
Extramammary Paget's disease	[154]	130	6	6	
	[155]	6	17	0	
	[156]	36	–	3	
	[157]	20	35	25	
	[158]	25	25	4	
Melanoma	[159]	19	26	18[b]	
	[160]	10	40	40	
	[161]	12	50	50	
	[162]	6	–	23[b]	
	[114]	61			75

[a]Progressive disease rate (1—objective response rate)
[b]5-year overall death rate

intermediate risk patients a 36% probability, and high risk patients an 80% probability. This risk categorization has been prospectively externally validated in a separate series of 37 patients [195].

The EAU guidelines panel for penile cancer updated the Solsona risk groups in their 2004 consensus document (Table 2.19) [19]. This categorization was externally validated and the probability of positive inguinal nodes was 4% for low risk, 35% for intermediate risk, and 46% for high risk patients [119]. Unfortunately, a more careful external validation of the Solsona and EAU risk groupings demonstrated that they had poor predictive accuracy (Table 2.19) [196]. The 2009 EAU guidelines on penile cancer have consequently dropped the risk groupings [197].

Gruppo Uro-Oncologico del Nord Est (GUONE) Nomogram

The first nomograms designed to predict penile cancer survival was the GUONE nomograms [198]. These nomograms were constructed using a moderately large penile cancer dataset consisting of the combined individual case series' of

Table 2.18 Molecular markers and penile cancer prognosis

Marker	References	Sample size	Percent positive (%)	Findings
Cell cycle regulation				
p53	[120]	43	40	No impact
	[182]	143	79	No correlation with HPV status
	[184]	86	42	↑ Nodes and ↓ survival
	[185]	297	–	↓ Survival
	[186]	52	58	No correlation with HPV status or outcome
	[187]	92	67	↓ Survival
	[188]	73	33	↑ Nodes and ↓ survival
	[189]	50		↓ Survival
p16[INK4A]	[120]	43	53	↑ Survival
	[182]	144	47	Positively correlated with HPV status
	[186]	52	50	Positively correlated with HPV status, ↓ nodes
	[190]	92	59	↑ Survival
p21	[182]	143	62	Positively correlated with HPV status
	[187]	92	33	No impact
RB	[182]	147	58	Negatively correlated with HPV status
Cyclin D1	[187]	92	42	No impact
MDM2	[185]	297	–	No impact
Cell proliferation				
Ki-67 (MIB-1)	[120]	43	86	No impact
	[188]	73	36	No impact
	[191]	117	53	↑ Nodes
PCNA	[192]	117	65	↑ Nodes
	[189]	50		No impact
Cell adhesion				
E-cadherin	[188]	73	45[a]	↑ Nodes and ↓ survival
	[193]	125	35[a]	↑ Nodes
Extracellular matrix regulators				
MMP-9	[188]	73	47	↓ Survival
	[193]	125	72	↓ Survival
MMP-2	[193]	125	26	No impact
Growth factors				
EGFR	[181]	100	26	↑ Stage and negative HPV correlation
HER3	[181]	96	86	↑ Stage, ↑ grade and positive HPV correlation
HER4	[181]	85	13	↑ Grade
Akt	[181]	101	40	↑ Grade
PTEN	[181]	94	39	↑ Grade

[a]Low expression of E-cadherin is a positive test result

several Italian collaborators. Several candidate variables were considered and bootstrap methods were used to correct for over-optimism. Two models were considered, one with clinical node staging (model 1) and one with pathological node staging (model 2). Model 2 performed slightly better than model 1 though neither has been externally validated.

Zini Risk Groups

Zini et al. used the SEER database to develop a prognostic tool [82]. The model is very simple using just stage and grade. The problem is that the version of disease stage that was modeled was SEER stage, a staging schema that is not widely used. SEER staging consists of three

Table 2.19 Solsona and EAU risk groups

	Solsona	EAU
Low risk	Ta	Ta
	Tis	Tis
	T1, grade 1	T1, grade 1
Intermediate risk	T1, grade ≥2	T1, grade 2
	T2	
High risk	≥T3	≥T2
		Grade 3/4

categories: localized, regional, and metastatic. Since most people use the TNM system, this model is unlikely to be used much and has not been externally validated.

Thuret Nomogram

The most recent penile cancer prognostic tool was proposed by Thuret et al. [199]. This tool is unique in that it predicts conditional cancer-specific survival, a survival outcome that takes into account the time between treatment and the current postoperative time-point. For example, imagine two penile cancer patients with identical disease features, one having had his surgery on January 1, 2008 and one on January 1, 2010. The 5-year conditional survival prediction will be different for these two patients, and the patient with the longer "surgery-to-present-time" interval will have a predicted survival outcome that is more favorable. This model has not been externally validated. Comparisons of the above penile prognostic tools are displayed in Table 2.20.

Conclusion

For penile carcinoma, many staging systems have been developed over time. Currently, the TNM classification is the most widely recognized and used staging methodology. However, even with the 2010 TNM update, there continues to be debate regarding the appropriate classification of penile cancer. Imaging plays a crucial role in enhancing the precision of clinical

staging and optimizing surgical planning. Recently, great improvements have been made in field of imaging which are affecting our ability to more precisely stage penile cancer. High resolution MRI now represents the gold standard for evaluating the primary tumor and its local extension. LNMRI and DSNB appear to be the superior modalities present for imaging regional lymph nodes. PET/CT has shown great promise as a whole body screen for the detection of distant metastases.

Patient prognosis is one of the most important factors considered in medical decision-making. Physicians tailor treatment recommendations based on expected survival and patients alter their willingness to accept treatment-associated risk when faced with different prognoses. The most basic prognosis that can be provided to a penile cancer patient is an unadjusted estimate of their expected survival. However, the outcomes of these patients depend not only on their diagnosis of penile cancer, but also on their overall state of health. For penile cancer, patient-related prognostic factors such as age, clinical/pathological stage, lymphovascular invasion, tumor grade and histology all impact survival. Prognostic tools, such as risk groupings and nomograms, which combine these individual factors, allow for a more precise estimate of patient outcomes. Few tools, such as those proposed by GUONE, Zini and Thuret, are available for penile cancer, but necessitate external validation prior to being incorporated into our medical decision-making armamentarium.

References

1. Baker BH, Watson FR. Staging carcinoma of the penis. J Surg Oncol. 1975;7(3):243–8.
2. Jackson SM. The treatment of carcinoma of the penis. Br J Surg. 1966;53(1):33–5.
3. Edge SB, Byrd DR, Compton CC, et al. AJCC: Penis AJCC cancer staging manual. 7th ed. New York: Springer; 2010. p. 447–55.
4. Slaton JW, Morgenstern N, Levy DA, Santos Jr MW, Tamboli P, Ro JY, et al. Tumor stage, vascular inva-

Table 2.20 Comparison of various penile cancer prognostic tools

	Solsona risk groups	EAU risk groups	GUONE nomograms	Zini	Thuret
References	[6]	[19]	[198]	[82]	[199]
Population	Italian Case series Single center	–	Italian Case series Multicenter	USA Population-based SEER	USA Population-based SEER
Development sample size	66	–	175	856	1,245
Variables in tool	T stage Grade	T stage Grade	Tumor thickness Growth pattern Grade LVI[a] Cavernosal inv.[b] Spongiosal inv. Urethral inv. Node status	SEER stage Grade	T stage N stage Grade
Tool type	Risk grouping	Risk grouping	Pictorial nomogram	Risk table	Pictorial nomogram
Predicted outcome	Positive lymph node rate	Positive lymph node rate	Cancer-specific survival	Cancer-specific survival	Conditional survival
Internal discrimination[c]	–	–	Model 1: 0.728 Model 2: 0.747	0.738	0.781
External discrimination	0.697	0.632	–	–	–
External validation	[195, 196]	[196]	–	–	–

[a]Lymphovascular invasion
[b]Invasion
[c]The measure of discrimination is Harrell's concordance index (i.e., area under the ROC curve)

sion and the percentage of poorly differentiated cancer: independent prognosticators for inguinal lymph node metastasis in penile squamous cancer. J Urol. 2001;165(4):1138–42.

5. McDougal WS. Carcinoma of the penis: improved survival by early regional lymphadenectomy based on the histological grade and depth of invasion of the primary lesion. J Urol. 1995;154(4):1364–6.

6. Solsona E, Iborra I, Ricos JV, Monros JL, Dumont R, Casanova J, et al. Corpus cavernosum invasion and tumor grade in the prediction of lymph node condition in penile carcinoma. Eur Urol. 1992;22(2): 115–8.

7. Soria JC, Fizazi K, Piron D, Kramar A, Gerbaulet A, Haie-Meder C, et al. Squamous cell carcinoma of the penis: multivariate analysis of prognostic factors and natural history in monocentric study with a conservative policy. Ann Oncol. 1997;8(11):1089–98.

8. Leijte JA, Gallee M, Antonini N, Horenblas S. Evaluation of current TNM classification of penile carcinoma. J Urol. 2008;180(3):933–8. discussion 8.

9. Leijte JA, Horenblas S. Shortcomings of the current TNM classification for penile carcinoma: time for a change? World J Urol. 2009;27(2):151–4.

10. Horenblas S, Van Tinteren H, Delemarre JF, Moonen LM, Lustig V, Kroger R. Squamous cell carcinoma of the penis: accuracy of tumor, nodes and metastasis classification system, and role of lymphangiography, computerized tomography scan and fine needle aspiration cytology. J Urol. 1991;146(5):1279–83.

11. Vapnek JM, Hricak H, Carroll PR. Recent advances in imaging studies for staging of penile and urethral carcinoma. Urol Clin North Am. 1992;19(2):257–66.

12. Sufrin G, Huben R. Benign and malignant lesions of the penis. In: Gillenwater JY, Grayhack JT, Howards SS, Mitchell ME, editors. Adult and pediatric urology. 4th ed. Philadelphia, PA: Lippincott Williams and Wilkins; 2002. p. 1975–2009.

13. Raghavaiah NV. Corpus cavernosogram in the evaluation of carcinoma of the penis. J Urol. 1978;120(4): 423–4.

14. Escribano G, Allona A, Burgos FJ, Garcia R, Navio S, Escudero A. Cavernosography in diagnosis of metastatic tumors of the penis: 5 new cases and a review of the literature. J Urol. 1987;138(5): 1174–7.

15. Haddad FS, Kovac A, Kivirand A, Sonkin B. Cavernosography in diagnosis of penile metastases secondary to bladder cancer. Urology. 1985;26(6): 585–6.

16. Agrawal A, Pai D, Ananthakrishnan N, Smile SR, Ratnakar C. Clinical and sonographic findings in carcinoma of the penis. J Clin Ultrasound. 2000;28(8): 399–406.

17. Bertolotto M, Serafini G, Dogliotti L, Gandolfo N, Gandolfo NG, Belgrano M, et al. Primary and secondary malignancies of the penis: ultrasound features. Abdom Imaging. 2005;30(1):108–12.

18. Horenblas S, Kroger R, Gallee MP, Newling DW, van Tinteren H. Ultrasound in squamous cell carci-

noma of the penis; a useful addition to clinical staging? A comparison of ultrasound with histopathology. Urology. 1994;43(5):702–7.

19. Solsona E, Algaba F, Horenblas S, Pizzocaro G, Windahl T. EAU guidelines on penile cancer. Eur Urol. 2004;46(1):1–8.

20. Kim B, Kawashima A, LeRoy AJ. Imaging of the male urethra. Semin Ultrasound CT MR. 2007;28(4): 258–73.

21. Ryu J, Kim B. MR imaging of the male and female urethra. Radiographics. 2001;21(5):1169–85.

22. Scher B, Seitz M, Reiser M, Hungerhuber E, Hahn K, Tiling R, et al. 18F-FDG PET/CT for staging of penile cancer. J Nucl Med. 2005;46(9):1460–5.

23. Kochhar R, Taylor B, Sangar V. Imaging in primary penile cancer: current status and future directions. Eur Radiol. 2010;20(1):36–47.

24. Pretorius ES, Siegelman ES, Ramchandani P, Banner MP. MR imaging of the penis. Radiographics. 2001;21 Spec No:S283–98; discussion S98–9.

25. Vossough A, Pretorius ES, Siegelman ES, Ramchandani P, Banner MP. Magnetic resonance imaging of the penis. Abdom Imaging. 2002;27(6): 640–59.

26. Petralia G, Villa G, Scardino E, Zoffoli E, Renne G, de Cobelli O, et al. Local staging of penile cancer using magnetic resonance imaging with pharmacologically induced penile erection. Radiol Med. 2008;113(4):517–28.

27. Scardino E, Villa G, Bonomo G, Matei DV, Verweij F, Rocco B, et al. Magnetic resonance imaging combined with artificial erection for local staging of penile cancer. Urology. 2004;63(6):1158–62.

28. Kayes O, Minhas S, Allen C, Hare C, Freeman A, Ralph D. The role of magnetic resonance imaging in the local staging of penile cancer. Eur Urol. 2007;51(5):1313–8. discussion 8–9.

29. Lorenzo AJ, Zimmern P, Lemack GE, Nurenberg P. Endorectal coil magnetic resonance imaging for diagnosis of urethral and periurethral pathologic findings in women. Urology. 2003;61(6):1129–33. discussion 33–4.

30. Macura KJ, Genadry R, Borman TL, Mostwin JL, Lardo AC, Bluemke DA. Evaluation of the female urethra with intraurethral magnetic resonance imaging. J Magn Reson Imaging. 2004;20(1):153–9.

31. Tan IL, Stoker J, Lameris JS. Magnetic resonance imaging of the female pelvic floor and urethra: body coil versus endovaginal coil. MAGMA. 1997;5(1): 59–63.

32. Blander DS, Rovner ES, Schnall MD, Ramchandani P, Banner MP, Broderick GA, et al. Endoluminal magnetic resonance imaging in the evaluation of urethral diverticula in women. Urology. 2001;57(4):660–5.

33. Singh AK, Saokar A, Hahn PF, Harisinghani MG. Imaging of penile neoplasms. Radiographics. 2005; 25(6):1629–38.

34. Mueller-Lisse UG, Scher B, Scherr MK, Seitz M. Functional imaging in penile cancer: PET/computed

tomography, MRI, and sentinel lymph node biopsy. Curr Opin Urol. 2008;18(1):105–10.

35. Hughes BE, Leijte JA, Kroon BK, Shabbir MA, Swallow TW, Heenan SD, et al. Lymph node metastasis in intermediate-risk penile squamous cell cancer: a two-centre experience. Eur Urol. 2010; 57(4):688–92.

36. Hungerhuber E, Schlenker B, Karl A, Frimberger D, Rothenberger KH, Stief CG, et al. Risk stratification in penile carcinoma: 25-year experience with surgical inguinal lymph node staging. Urology. 2006; 68(3):621–5.

37. Kroon BK, Horenblas S, Lont AP, Tanis PJ, Gallee MP, Nieweg OE. Patients with penile carcinoma benefit from immediate resection of clinically occult lymph node metastases. J Urol. 2005;173(3):816–9.

38. Sufrin G, Huben R. Benign and malignant lesions of the penis. In: Gillenwater JY, Grayhack JT, Howards SS, Michell ME, editors. Adult and pediatric urology. 4th ed. Philadelphia, PA: Lippincott Williams and Wilkins; 2002. p. 1975–2009.

39. Bouchot O, Rigaud J, Maillet F, Hetet JF, Karam G. Morbidity of inguinal lymphadenectomy for invasive penile carcinoma. Eur Urol. 2004;45(6):761–5. discussion 5–6.

40. Esen G. Ultrasound of superficial lymph nodes. Eur J Radiol. 2006;58(3):345–59.

41. Steinkamp HJ, Mueffelmann M, Bock JC, Thiel T, Kenzel P, Felix R. Differential diagnosis of lymph node lesions: a semiquantitative approach with colour Doppler ultrasound. Br J Radiol. 1998;71(848):828–33.

42. Crawshaw JW, Hadway P, Hoffland D, Bassingham S, Corbishley CM, Smith Y, et al. Sentinel lymph node biopsy using dynamic lymphoscintigraphy combined with ultrasound-guided fine needle aspiration in penile carcinoma. Br J Radiol. 2009;82(973):41–8.

43. Hall TB, Barton DP, Trott PA, Nasiri N, Shepherd JH, Thomas JM, et al. The role of ultrasound-guided cytology of groin lymph nodes in the management of squamous cell carcinoma of the vulva: 5-year experience in 44 patients. Clin Radiol. 2003;58(5):367–71.

44. Kroon BK, Horenblas S, Deurloo EE, Nieweg OE, Teertstra HJ. Ultrasonography-guided fine-needle aspiration cytology before sentinel node biopsy in patients with penile carcinoma. BJU Int. 2005;95(4):517–21.

45. Lont AP, Besnard AP, Gallee MP, van Tinteren H, Horenblas S. A comparison of physical examination and imaging in determining the extent of primary penile carcinoma. BJU Int. 2003;91(6):493–5.

46. Graafland NM, Leijte JA, Valdes Olmos RA, Hoefnagel CA, Teertstra HJ, Horenblas S. Scanning with 18F-FDG-PET/CT for detection of pelvic nodal involvement in inguinal node-positive penile carcinoma. Eur Urol. 2009;56(2):339–45.

47. Kitajima K, Murakami K, Yamasaki E, Fukasawa I, Inaba N, Kaji Y, et al. Accuracy of 18F-FDG PET/CT in detecting pelvic and paraaortic lymph node metastasis in patients with endometrial cancer. AJR Am J Roentgenol. 2008;190(6):1652–8.

48. Ng SH, Yen TC, Chang JT, Chan SC, Ko SF, Wang HM, et al. Prospective study of [18F] fluorodeoxyglucose positron emission tomography and computed tomography and magnetic resonance imaging in oral cavity squamous cell carcinoma with palpably negative neck. J Clin Oncol. 2006;24(27): 4371–6.

49. Leijte JA, Graafland NM, Valdes Olmos RA, van Boven HH, Hoefnagel CA, Horenblas S. Prospective evaluation of hybrid 18F-fluorodeoxyglucose positron emission tomography/computed tomography in staging clinically node-negative patients with penile carcinoma. BJU Int. 2009;104(5):640–4.

50. Tabatabaei S, Harisinghani M, McDougal WS. Regional lymph node staging using lymphotropic nanoparticle enhanced magnetic resonance imaging with ferumoxtran-10 in patients with penile cancer. J Urol. 2005;174(3):923–7. discussion 7.

51. Kroon BK, Nieweg OE, van Boven H, Horenblas S. Size of metastasis in the sentinel node predicts additional nodal involvement in penile carcinoma. J Urol. 2006;176(1):105–8.

52. Thoeny HC, Triantafyllou M, Birkhaeuser FD, Froehlich JM, Tshering DW, Binser T, et al. Combined ultrasmall superparamagnetic particles of iron oxide-enhanced and diffusion-weighted magnetic resonance imaging reliably detect pelvic lymph node metastases in normal-sized nodes of bladder and prostate cancer patients. Eur Urol. 2009; 55(4):761–9.

53. Morton DL, Cochran AJ, Thompson JF, Elashoff R, Essner R, Glass EC, et al. Sentinel node biopsy for early-stage melanoma: accuracy and morbidity in MSLT-I, an international multicenter trial. Ann Surg. 2005;242(3):302–11. discussion 11–3.

54. Gonzaga-Silva LF, Tavares JM, Freitas FC, Tomas Filho ME, Oliveira VP, Lima MV. The isolated gamma probe technique for sentinel node penile carcinoma detection is unreliable. Int Braz J Urol. 2007;33(1):58–63. discussion 4–7.

55. Spiess PE, Izawa JI, Bassett R, Kedar D, Busby JE, Wong F, et al. Preoperative lymphoscintigraphy and dynamic sentinel node biopsy for staging penile cancer: results with pathological correlation. J Urol. 2007;177(6):2157–61.

56. Tanis PJ, Lont AP, Meinhardt W, Olmos RA, Nieweg OE, Horenblas S. Dynamic sentinel node biopsy for penile cancer: reliability of a staging technique. J Urol. 2002;168(1):76–80.

57. Hegarty PK, Minhas S. Re: Evaluation of dynamic lymphoscintigraphy and sentinel lymph-node biopsy for detecting occult metastases in patients with penile squamous cell carcinoma. BJU Int. 2008; 101(6):781. author reply 781–2.

58. Horenblas S. Words of wisdom. Re: Preoperative lymphoscintigraphy and dynamic sentinel node biopsy for staging penile cancer: results with pathological correlation. Eur Urol. 2007;52(4):1261.

59. Leijte JA, Kroon BK, Valdes Olmos RA, Nieweg OE, Horenblas S. Reliability and safety of current dynamic sentinel node biopsy for penile carcinoma. Eur Urol. 2007;52(1):170–7.

60. Leijte JA, Hughes B, Graafland NM, Kroon BK, Olmos RA, Nieweg OE, et al. Two-center evaluation of dynamic sentinel node biopsy for squamous cell carcinoma of the penis. J Clin Oncol. 2009;27(20): 3325–9.

61. Jeffrey C, Applewhite MCH, McCullough DL. Urethral carcinoma. In: Gillenwater JY, Grayhack JT, Howards SS, Mitchell ME, editors. Adult and pediatric urology. 4th ed. Philadelphia, PA: Lippincott Williams and Wilkins; 2002. p. 1791–810.

62. Poeppel TD, Krause BJ, Heusner TA, Boy C, Bockisch A, Antoch G. PET/CT for the staging and follow-up of patients with malignancies. Eur J Radiol. 2009;70(3):382–92.

63. Krabbe CA, Pruim J, van der Laan BF, Rodiger LA, Roodenburg JL. FDG-PET and detection of distant metastases and simultaneous tumors in head and neck squamous cell carcinoma: a comparison with chest radiography and chest CT. Oral Oncol. 2009;45(3):234–40.

64. Gourin CG, Watts T, Williams HT, Patel VS, Bilodeau PA, Coleman TA. Identification of distant metastases with PET-CT in patients with suspected recurrent head and neck cancer. Laryngoscope. 2009;119(4):703–6.

65. Hagerty RG, Butow PN, Ellis PM, Dimitry S, Tattersall MH. Communicating prognosis in cancer care: a systematic review of the literature. Ann Oncol. 2005;16(7):1005–53.

66. Maddineni SB, Lau MM, Sangar VK. Identifying the needs of penile cancer sufferers: a systematic review of the quality of life, psychosexual and psychosocial literature in penile cancer. BMC Urol. 2009;9:8.

67. Meredith C, Symonds P, Webster L, Lamont D, Pyper E, Gillis CR, et al. Information needs of cancer patients in west Scotland: cross sectional survey of patients' views. BMJ. 1996;313(7059):724–6.

68. Kaplowitz SA, Campo S, Chiu WT. Cancer patients' desires for communication of prognosis information. Health Commun. 2002;14(2):221–41.

69. Kleinbaum DG, Morgenstern H, Kupper LL. Selection bias in epidemiologic studies. Am J Epidemiol. 1981;113(4):452–63.

70. Antman K, Amato D, Wood W, Carson J, Suit H, Proppe K, et al. Selection bias in clinical trials. J Clin Oncol. 1985;3(8):1142–7.

71. Miller KD, Rahman ZU, Sledge Jr GW. Selection bias in clinical trials. Breast Dis. 2001;14:31–40.

72. Grimes DA, Schulz KF. Bias and causal associations in observational research. Lancet. 2002;359(9302): 248–52.

73. Justice AC, Covinsky KE, Berlin JA. Assessing the generalizability of prognostic information. Ann Intern Med. 1999;130(6):515–24.

74. Izquierdo JN, Schoenbach VJ. The potential and limitations of data from population-based state cancer registries. Am J Public Health. 2000;90(5):695–8.

75. Siegel R, Naishadham D, Jemal A. Cancer statistics, 2012. CA Cancer J Clin. 2012;62(1):10–29 [Comparative Study].

76. Rothman KJ, Greenland S, Lash TL. Modern epidemiology. 3rd ed. Philadephia, PA: Lippincott Williams and Wilkins; 2008.

77. Collett D. Modelling survival data in medical research. 2nd ed. Boca Raton, FL: Chapman & Hall/ CRC; 2003.

78. dos Santos SI. Cancer epidemiology: principles and methods. Lyon: International Agency for Research on Cancer; 1999.

79. Welch HG, Black WC. Are deaths within 1 month of cancer-directed surgery attributed to cancer? J Natl Cancer Inst. 2002;94(14):1066–70.

80. Gooley TA, Leisenring W, Crowley J, Storer BE. Estimation of failure probabilities in the presence of competing risks: new representations of old estimators. Stat Med. 1999;18(6):695–706.

81. Pintilie M. Competing risks: a practical perspective. Hoboken, NJ: Wiley; 2006.

82. Zini L, Cloutier V, Isbarn H, Perrotte P, Capitanio U, Jeldres C, et al. A simple and accurate model for prediction of cancer-specific mortality in patients treated with surgery for primary penile squamous cell carcinoma. Clin Cancer Res. 2009;15(3):1013–8.

83. Gamel JW, Vogel RL. Non-parametric comparison of relative versus cause-specific survival in surveillance, epidemiology and end results (SEER) programme breast cancer patients. Stat Methods Med Res. 2001;10(5):339–52.

84. Ederer F, Axtell LM, Cutler SJ. The relative survival rate: a statistical methodology. Natl Cancer Inst Monogr. 1961;6:101–21.

85. Ederer F, Heise H. Instructions to IBM 650 programmers in processing survival computations. Methodological note no. 10. In: Natl Cancer Inst Monogr, editor. End results evaluation section NCI. Bethesda, MD: Natl Cancer Inst Monogr; 1959.

86. Hakulinen T. Cancer survival corrected for heterogeneity in patient withdrawal. Biometrics. 1982;38(4): 933–42.

87. Dickman PW, Adami HO. Interpreting trends in cancer patient survival. J Intern Med. 2006;260(2): 103–17.

88. Verhoeven RHA. Epidemiology of uncommon male genital cancers. Studies with regional, national and international cancer registry data. Erasmus Universiteit Rotterdam: Optima Grafische Communicatie; 2012.

89. Verhoeven RHA, Gondos A, Janssen-Heijnen MLG, Zanetti R, Caldarella A, Brewster DH, et al. Population-based survival of penile cancer patients in Europe and the USA since 1990. 3rd European Multidisciplinary Meeting on Urological Cancers; Barcelona, Spain; 2011.

90. Engholm G, Ferlay J, Christensen N, Bray F, Gjerstorff ML, Klint A, et al. NORDCAN—a Nordic tool for cancer information, planning, quality control and research. Acta Oncol. 2010;49(5):725–36.

91. Graafland NM, Verhoeven RH, Coebergh JW, Horenblas S. Incidence trends and survival of penile squamous cell carcinoma in the Netherlands. Int J Cancer. 2011;128(2):426–32.

92. Service SWPHOfNCI. Penile cancer incidence, mortality and survival rates in England: summary. 2010 [cited 2012 5/29/2012]. Available from: www.swpho.nhs.uk/urologicalcancerhub/view.aspx?rid=92.

93. Visser O, Adolfsson J, Rossi S, Verne J, Gatta G, Maffezzini M, et al. Incidence and survival of rare urogenital cancers in Europe. Eur J Cancer. 2012;48(4):456–64 [Research Support, Non-U.S. Gov't].

94. Bray F, Klint A, Gislum M, Hakulinen T, Engholm G, Tryggvadottir L, et al. Trends in survival of patients diagnosed with male genital cancers in the Nordic countries 1964–2003 followed up until the end of 2006. Acta Oncol. 2010;49(5):644–54.

95. Ghani AC, Donnelly CA, Cox DR, Griffin JT, Fraser C, Lam TH, et al. Methods for estimating the case fatality ratio for a novel, emerging infectious disease. Am J Epidemiol. 2005;162(5):479–86.

96. Morrison BF, Hanchard B, Graham RP, Reid ME. Penile cancer in Jamaicans managed at the University Hospital of the West Indies. West Indian Med J. 2011;60(5):525–30.

97. Blank TO, Bellizzi KM. A gerontologic perspective on cancer and aging. Cancer. 2008;112(11 Suppl):2569–76 [Review].

98. Kirchberger I, Meisinger C, Heier M, Zimmermann AK, Thorand B, Autenrieth CS, et al. Patterns of multimorbidity in the aged population. Results from the KORA-Age study. PLoS One. 2012;7(1):e30556.

99. Marengoni A, Angleman S, Melis R, Mangialasche F, Karp A, Garmen A, et al. Aging with multimorbidity: a systematic review of the literature. Ageing Res Rev. 2011;10(4):430–9.

100. van den Akker M, Buntinx F, Metsemakers JF, Roos S, Knottnerus JA. Multimorbidity in general practice: prevalence, incidence, and determinants of co-occurring chronic and recurrent diseases. J Clin Epidemiol. 1998;51(5):367–75.

101. Yellen SB, Cella DF, Leslie WT. Age and clinical decision making in oncology patients. J Natl Cancer Inst. 1994;86(23):1766–70.

102. Wedding U, Honecker F, Bokemeyer C, Pientka L, Hoffken K. Tolerance to chemotherapy in elderly patients with cancer. Cancer Control. 2007;14(1):44–56 [Research Support, Non-U.S. Gov't Review].

103. Muss HB, Berry DA, Cirrincione C, Budman DR, Henderson IC, Citron ML, et al. Toxicity of older and younger patients treated with adjuvant chemotherapy for node-positive breast cancer: the Cancer and Leukemia Group B Experience. J Clin Oncol. 2007;25(24):3699–704 [Randomized Controlled Trial Research Support, N.I.H., Extramural].

104. Foster JA, Salinas GD, Mansell D, Williamson JC, Casebeer LL. How does older age influence oncologists' cancer management? Oncologist. 2010;15(6):584–92.

105. Meza R, Jeon J, Moolgavkar SH, Luebeck EG. Age-specific incidence of cancer: phases, transitions, and biological implications. Proc Natl Acad Sci U S A. 2008;105(42):16284–9.

106. Rao AV, Valk PJ, Metzeler KH, Acharya CR, Tuchman SA, Stevenson MM, et al. Age-specific differences in oncogenic pathway dysregulation and anthracycline sensitivity in patients with acute myeloid leukemia. J Clin Oncol. 2009;27(33):5580–6.

107. Hernandez BY, Barnholtz-Sloan J, German RR, Giuliano A, Goodman MT, King JB, et al. Burden of invasive squamous cell carcinoma of the penis in the United States, 1998–2003. Cancer. 2008;113(10 Suppl):2883–91.

108. Asadzadeh Vostakolaei F, Karim-Kos HE, Janssen-Heijnen ML, Visser O, Verbeek AL, Kiemeney LA. The validity of the mortality to incidence ratio as a proxy for site-specific cancer survival. Eur J Public Health. 2011;21(5):573–7.

109. Baldur-Felskov B, Hannibal CG, Munk C, Kjaer SK. Increased incidence of penile cancer and high-grade penile intraepithelial neoplasia in Denmark 1978–2008: a nationwide population-based study. Cancer Causes Control. 2012;23(2):273–80.

110. Barnholtz-Sloan JS, Maldonado JL, Pow-sang J, Giuliano AR. Incidence trends in primary malignant penile cancer. Urol Oncol. 2007;25(5):361–7.

111. Menotti A, Mulder I, Nissinen A, Giampaoli S, Feskens EJ, Kromhout D. Prevalence of morbidity and multimorbidity in elderly male populations and their impact on 10-year all-cause mortality: the FINE study (Finland, Italy, Netherlands, elderly). J Clin Epidemiol. 2001;54(7):680–6.

112. Ornellas AA, Seixas ALC, Marota A, Wisnescky A, Campos F, De Moraes JR. Surgical treatment of invasive squamous cell carcinoma of the penis: retrospective analysis of 350 cases. J Urol. 1994;151(5):1244–9.

113. Rippentrop JM, Joslyn SA, Konety BR. Squamous cell carcinoma of the penis: evaluation of data from the surveillance, epidemiology, and end results program. Cancer. 2004;101(6):1357–63.

114. Surveillance Epidemiology and End Results (SEER) Program (www.seer.cancer.gov). SEER*Stat Database: Incidence—SEER 18 Regs Research Data + Hurricane Katrina Impacted Louisiana Cases, Nov 2011 Sub (1973–2009 varying)—Linked To County Attributes—Total U.S., 1969–2010 Counties. In: National Cancer Institute D, Surveillance Research Program, Surveillance Systems Branch, editor.

115. Breslow A. Thickness, cross-sectional areas and depth of invasion in the prognosis of cutaneous melanoma. Ann Surg. 1970;172(5):902–8.

116. Edge SB, Byrd DR, Compton CC, Fritz AG, Greene FL, Trotti A, editors. AJCC cancer staging handbook. 7th ed. New York: Springer; 2010.

117. Clark Jr WH, From L, Bernardino EA, Mihm MC. The histogenesis and biologic behavior of primary human malignant melanomas of the skin. Cancer Res. 1969;29(3):705–27.

118. Dai B, Ye DW, Kong YY, Yao XD, Zhang HL, Shen YJ. Predicting regional lymph node metastasis in Chinese patients with penile squamous cell carcinoma: the role of histopathological classification, tumor stage and depth of invasion. J Urol. 2006;176(4 Pt 1):1431–5. discussion 5.

119. Ficarra V, Zattoni F, Cunico SC, Galetti TP, Luciani L, Fandella A, et al. Lymphatic and vascular embolizations are independent predictive variables of inguinal lymph node involvement in patients with squamous cell carcinoma of the penis: Gruppo Uro-Oncologico del Nord Est (Northeast Uro-Oncological Group) Penile Cancer data base data. Cancer. 2005;103(12):2507–16.

120. Bethune G, Campbell J, Rocker A, Bell D, Rendon R, Merrimen J. Clinical and pathologic factors of prognostic significance in penile squamous cell carcinoma in a North American population. Urology. 2012;79(5):1092–7.

121. Lopes A, Hidalgo GS, Kowalski LP, Torloni H, Rossi BM, Fonseca FP. Prognostic factors in carcinoma of the penis: multivariate analysis of 145 patients treated with amputation and lymphadenectomy. J Urol. 1996;156(5):1637–42.

122. Ornellas AA, Nobrega BL, Wei Kin Chin E, Wisnescky A, da Silva PC, de Santos Schwindt AB. Prognostic factors in invasive squamous cell carcinoma of the penis: analysis of 196 patients treated at the Brazilian National Cancer Institute. J Urol. 2008;180(4):1354–9.

123. Graafland NM, van Boven HH, van Werkhoven E, Moonen LM, Horenblas S. Prognostic significance of extranodal extension in patients with pathological node positive penile carcinoma. J Urol. 2010;184(4):1347–53.

124. Pandey D, Mahajan V, Kannan RR. Prognostic factors in node-positive carcinoma of the penis. J Surg Oncol. 2006;93(2):133–8.

125. Svatek RS, Munsell M, Kincaid JM, Hegarty P, Slaton JW, Busby JE, et al. Association between lymph node density and disease specific survival in patients with penile cancer. J Urol. 2009;182(6):2721–7.

126. Ornellas AA, Kinchin EW, Nobrega BL, Wisnescky A, Koifman N, Quirino R. Surgical treatment of invasive squamous cell carcinoma of the penis: Brazilian National Cancer Institute long-term experience. J Surg Oncol. 2008;97(6):487–95.

127. Gulia AK, Mandhani A, Muruganandham K, Kapoor R, Ansari MS, Srivastava A. Impact of delay in inguinal lymph node dissection in patients with carcinoma of penis. Indian J Cancer. 2009;46(3):214–8.

128. Marconnet L, Rigaud J, Bouchot O. Long-term followup of penile carcinoma with high risk for lymph node invasion treated with inguinal lymphadenectomy. J Urol. 2010;183(6):2227–32.

129. Pow-Sang MR, Benavente V, Pow-Sang JE, Morante C, Meza L, Baker M, et al. Cancer of the penis. Cancer Control. 2002;9(4):305–14.

130. Novara G, Galfano A, De Marco V, Artibani W, Ficarra V. Prognostic factors in squamous cell carcinoma of the penis. Nat Clin Pract Urol. 2007; 4(3):140–6.

131. Bolenz C, Fernandez MI, Tilki D, Herrmann E, Heinzelbecker J, Ergun S, et al. The role of lymphangiogenesis in lymphatic tumour spread of urological cancers. BJU Int. 2009;104(5):592–7.

132. Naumann CM, Al-Najar A, Alkatout I, Hegele A, Korda JB, Bolenz C, et al. Lymphatic spread in squamous cell carcinoma of the penis is independent of elevated lymph vessel density. BJU Int. 2009; 103(12):1655–9. discussion 9.

133. Guimaraes GC, Cunha IW, Soares FA, Lopes A, Torres J, Chaux A, et al. Penile squamous cell carcinoma clinicopathological features, nodal metastasis and outcome in 333 cases. J Urol. 2009;182(2):528–34. discussion 34.

134. Velazquez EF, Ayala G, Liu H, Chaux A, Zanotti M, Torres J, et al. Histologic grade and perineural invasion are more important than tumor thickness as predictor of nodal metastasis in penile squamous cell carcinoma invading 5 to 10 mm. Am J Surg Pathol. 2008;32(7):974–9.

135. Liebig C, Ayala G, Wilks JA, Berger DH, Albo D. Perineural invasion in cancer: a review of the literature. Cancer. 2009;115(15):3379–91 [Review].

136. Chaux A, Caballero C, Soares F, Guimaraes GC, Cunha IW, Reuter V, et al. The prognostic index: a useful pathologic guide for prediction of nodal metastases and survival in penile squamous cell carcinoma. Am J Surg Pathol. 2009;33(7):1049–57.

137. Leijte JA, Kirrander P, Antonini N, Windahl T, Horenblas S. Recurrence patterns of squamous cell carcinoma of the penis: recommendations for follow-up based on a two-centre analysis of 700 patients. Eur Urol. 2008;54(1):161–8.

138. Haas GP, Blumenstein BA, Gagliano RG, Russell CA, Rivkin SE, Culkin DJ, et al. Cisplatin, methotrexate and bleomycin for the treatment of carcinoma of the penis: a Southwest Oncology Group study. J Urol. 1999;161(6):1823–5.

139. Di Lorenzo G, Federico P, Buonerba C, Longo N, Carten G, Autorino R, et al. Paclitaxel in pretreated metastatic penile cancer: final results of a phase 2 study. Eur Urol. 2011;60(6):1280–4.

140. Ritchie AWS, Foster PW, Fowler S. Penile cancer in the UK: clinical presentation and outcome in 1998/99. BJU Int. 2004;94(9):1248–52.

141. Broders AC. Squamous-cell epithelioma of the lip: a study of five hundred and thirty-seven cases. JAMA. 1920;74(10):656–64.

142. Chaux A, Torres J, Pfannl R, Barreto J, Rodriguez I, Velazquez EF, et al. Histologic grade in penile squamous cell carcinoma: visual estimation versus digital measurement of proportions of grades, adverse prognosis with any proportion of grade 3

and correlation of a Gleason-like system with nodal metastasis. Am J Surg Pathol. 2009;33(7):1042–8.

143. Kamat MR, Kulkarni JN, Tongaonkar HB. Carcinoma of the penis: the Indian experience. J Surg Oncol. 1993;52(1):50–5.

144. Tyson MD, Etzioni DA, Wisenbaugh ES, Andrews PE, Humphreys MR, Ferrigni RG, et al. Anatomic site-specific disparities in survival outcomes for penile squamous cell carcinoma. Urology. 2012; 79(4):804–8.

145. Buschke A, Lowenstein L. Über carcinomahnliche condylomata acuminata des penis. Klin Wochenschr. 1925;4:1726–8.

146. Eble JN, Sauter G, Epstein JI, Sesterhenn IA, editors. World Health Organization classification of tumours. Pathology and genetics of tumours of the urinary system and male genital organs. Lyon: IARC; 2004.

147. Cubilla AL, Reuter VE, Gregoire L, Ayala G, Ocampos S, Lancaster WD, et al. Basaloid squamous cell carcinoma: a distinctive human papilloma virus-related penile neoplasm: a report of 20 cases. Am J Surg Pathol. 1998;22(6):755–61.

148. Velazquez EF, Melamed J, Barreto JE, Aguero F, Cubilla AL. Sarcomatoid carcinoma of the penis: a clinicopathologic study of 15 cases. Am J Surg Pathol. 2005;29(9):1152–8.

149. Lont AP, Gallee MP, Snijders P, Horenblas S. Sarcomatoid squamous cell carcinoma of the penis: a clinical and pathological study of 5 cases. J Urol. 2004;172(3):932–5.

150. Caccialanza M, Marca S, Piccinno R, Eulisse G. Radiotherapy of classic and human immunodeficiency virus-related Kaposi's sarcoma: results in 1482 lesions. J Eur Acad Dermatol Venereol. 2008;22(3): 297–302.

151. Kirova YM, Belembaogo E, Frikha H, Haddad E, Calitchi E, Levy E, et al. Radiotherapy in the management of epidemic Kaposi's sarcoma: a retrospective study of 643 cases. Radiother Oncol. 1998;46(1):19–22.

152. Fetsch JF, Davis Jr CJ, Miettinen M, Sesterhenn IA. Leiomyosarcoma of the penis: a clinicopathologic study of 14 cases with review of the literature and discussion of the differential diagnosis. Am J Surg Pathol. 2004;28(1):115–25.

153. Dominici A, Delle Rose A, Stomaci N, Pugliese L, Posti A, Nesi G. A rare case of leiomyosarcoma of the penis with a reappraisal of the literature. Int J Urol. 2004;11(6):440–4.

154. Wang Z, Lu M, Dong GQ, Jiang YQ, Lin MS, Cai ZK, et al. Penile and Scrotal Paget's disease: 130 Chinese patients with long-term follow-up. BJU Int. 2008;102(4):485–8.

155. Park S, Grossfeld GD, McAninch JW, Santucci R. Extramammary Paget's disease of the penis and scrotum: excision, reconstruction and evaluation of occult malignancy. J Urol. 2001;166(6):2112–6. discussion 7.

156. Yang WJ, Kim DS, Im YJ, Cho KS, Rha KH, Cho NH, et al. Extramammary Paget's disease of penis and scrotum. Urology. 2005;65(5):972–5.

157. Hegarty PK, Suh J, Fisher MB, Taylor J, Nguyen TH, Ivan D, et al. Penoscrotal extramammary Paget's disease: the University of Texas M.D. Anderson Cancer Center contemporary experience. J Urol. 2011;186(1):97–102.

158. Zhang N, Gong K, Zhang X, Yang Y, Na Y. Extramammary Paget's disease of scrotum—report of 25 cases and literature review. Urol Oncol. 2010;28(1):28–33.

159. van Geel AN, den Bakker MA, Kirkels W, Horenblas S, Kroon BB, de Wilt JH, et al. Prognosis of primary mucosal penile melanoma: a series of 19 Dutch patients and 47 patients from the literature. Urology. 2007;70(1):143–7.

160. Sanchez-Ortiz R, Huang SF, Tamboli P, Prieto VG, Hester G, Pettaway CA. Melanoma of the penis, scrotum and male urethra: a 40-year single institution experience. J Urol. 2005;173(6):1958–65.

161. Oxley JD, Corbishley C, Down L, Watkin N, Dickerson D, Wong NA. Clinicopathological and molecular study of penile melanoma. J Clin Pathol. 2012;65(3):228–31.

162. Larsson KB, Shaw HM, Thompson JF, Harman RC, McCarthy WH. Primary mucosal and glans penis melanomas: the Sydney Melanoma Unit experience. Aust N Z J Surg. 1999;69(2):121–6.

163. Centre. WIICoHaCCHI. WHO/ICO Information Centre on HPV and Cervical Cancer (HPV Information Centre). Human Papillomavirus and Related Cancers in World. Summary Report 2010. Available at www. who. int/ hpvcentre 2010;2010.

164. Backes DM, Kurman RJ, Pimenta JM, Smith JS. Systematic review of human papillomavirus prevalence in invasive penile cancer. Cancer Causes Control. 2009;20(4):449–57.

165. Kirrander P, Kolaric A, Helenius G, Windahl T, Andren O, Stark JR, et al. Human papillomavirus prevalence, distribution and correlation to histopathological parameters in a large Swedish cohort of men with penile carcinoma. BJU Int. 2011;108(3):355–9.

166. Dayyani F, Etzel CJ, Liu M, Ho CH, Lippman SM, Tsao AS. Meta-analysis of the impact of human papillomavirus (HPV) on cancer risk and overall survival in head and neck squamous cell carcinomas (HNSCC). Head Neck Oncol. 2010;2:15.

167. Gillison ML, Koch WM, Capone RB, Spafford M, Westra WH, Wu L, et al. Evidence for a causal association between human papillomavirus and a subset of head and neck cancers. J Natl Cancer Inst. 2000;92(9):709–20.

168. Kreimer AR, Clifford GM, Boyle P, Franceschi S. Human papillomavirus types in head and neck squamous cell carcinomas worldwide: a systematic review. Cancer Epidemiol Biomarkers Prev. 2005;14(2):467–75.

169. Fakhry C, Westra WH, Li S, Cmelak A, Ridge JA, Pinto H, et al. Improved survival of patients with

human papillomavirus-positive head and neck squamous cell carcinoma in a prospective clinical trial. J Natl Cancer Inst. 2008;100(4):261–9.

170. Ragin CC, Taioli E. Survival of squamous cell carcinoma of the head and neck in relation to human papillomavirus infection: review and meta-analysis. Int J Cancer. 2007;121(8):1813–20.

171. Rautava J, Kuuskoski J, Syrjanen K, Grenman R, Syrjanen S. HPV genotypes and their prognostic significance in head and neck squamous cell carcinomas. J Clin Virol. 2012;53(2):116–20.

172. Gillison ML, D'Souza G, Westra W, Sugar E, Xiao W, Begum S, et al. Distinct risk factor profiles for human papillomavirus type 16-positive and human papillomavirus type 16-negative head and neck cancers. J Natl Cancer Inst. 2008;100(6):407–20.

173. Smith EM, Wang D, Kim Y, Rubenstein LM, Lee JH, Haugen TH, et al. P16INK4a expression, human papillomavirus, and survival in head and neck cancer. Oral Oncol. 2008;44(2):133–42.

174. Scheiner MA, Campos MM, Ornellas AA, Chin EW, Ornellas MH, Andrada-Serpa MJ. Human papillomavirus and penile cancers in Rio de Janeiro, Brazil: HPV typing and clinical features. Int Braz J Urol. 2008;34(4):467–74. discussion 75–6.

175. Bezerra AL, Lopes A, Santiago GH, Ribeiro KC, Latorre MR, Villa LL. Human papillomavirus as a prognostic factor in carcinoma of the penis: analysis of 82 patients treated with amputation and bilateral lymphadenectomy. Cancer. 2001;91(12): 2315–21.

176. Gregoire L, Cubilla AL, Reuter VE, Haas GP, Lancaster WD. Preferential association of human papillomavirus with high-grade histologic variants of penile-invasive squamous cell carcinoma. J Natl Cancer Inst. 1995;87(22):1705–9.

177. Krustrup D, Jensen HL, van den Brule AJ, Frisch M. Histological characteristics of human papillomavirus-positive and -negative invasive and in situ squamous cell tumours of the penis. Int J Exp Pathol. 2009;90(2):182–9.

178. Lont AP, Kroon BK, Horenblas S, Gallee MP, Berkhof J, Meijer CJ, et al. Presence of high-risk human papillomavirus DNA in penile carcinoma predicts favorable outcome in survival. Int J Cancer. 2006;119(5):1078–81.

179. Miralles-Guri C, Bruni L, Cubilla AL, Castellsague X, Bosch FX, de Sanjose S. Human papillomavirus prevalence and type distribution in penile carcinoma. J Clin Pathol. 2009;62(10):870–8.

180. Rubin MA, Kleter B, Zhou M, Ayala G, Cubilla AL, Quint WG, et al. Detection and typing of human papillomavirus DNA in penile carcinoma: evidence for multiple independent pathways of penile carcinogenesis. Am J Pathol. 2001;159(4):1211–8.

181. Stankiewicz E, Prowse DM, Ng M, Cuzick J, Mesher D, Hiscock F, et al. Alternative HER/PTEN/Akt pathway activation in HPV positive and negative penile carcinomas. PLoS One. 2011;6(3):e17517.

182. Stankiewicz E, Prowse DM, Ktori E, Cuzick J, Ambroisine L, Zhang X, et al. The retinoblastoma protein/p16 INK4A pathway but not p53 is disrupted by human papillomavirus in penile squamous cell carcinoma. Histopathology. 2011;58(3):433–9.

183. Giuliano AR, Palefsky JM, Goldstone S, Moreira Jr ED, Penny ME, Aranda C, et al. Efficacy of quadrivalent HPV vaccine against HPV Infection and disease in males. N Engl J Med. 2011;364(5):401–11 [Multicenter Study Randomized Controlled Trial Research Support, N.I.H., Extramural Research Support, Non-U.S. Gov't].

184. Lopes A, Bezerra AL, Pinto CA, Serrano SV, de Mell OC, Villa LL. p53 as a new prognostic factor for lymph node metastasis in penile carcinoma: analysis of 82 patients treated with amputation and bilateral lymphadenectomy. J Urol. 2002;168(1):81–6.

185. Rocha RM, Ignacio JA, Jordan J, Carraro DM, Lisboa B, Lopes A, et al. A clinical, pathologic, and molecular study of p53 and murine double minute 2 in penile carcinogenesis and its relation to prognosis. Hum Pathol. 2012;43(4):481–8.

186. Poetsch M, Hemmerich M, Kakies C, Kleist B, Wolf E, vom Dorp F, et al. Alterations in the tumor suppressor gene p16(INK4A) are associated with aggressive behavior of penile carcinomas. Virchows Arch. 2011;458(2):221–9.

187. Gunia S, Kakies C, Erbersdobler A, Hakenberg OW, Koch S, May M. Expression of p53, p21 and cyclin D1 in penile cancer: p53 predicts poor prognosis. J Clin Pathol. 2012;65(3):232–6.

188. Zhu Y, Zhou XY, Yao XD, Dai B, Ye DW. The prognostic significance of p53, Ki-67, epithelial cadherin and matrix metalloproteinase-9 in penile squamous cell carcinoma treated with surgery. BJU Int. 2007; 100(1):204–8.

189. Martins AC, Faria SM, Cologna AJ, Suaid HJ, Tucci Jr S. Immunoexpression of p53 protein and proliferating cell nuclear antigen in penile carcinoma. J Urol. 2002;167(1):89–92. discussion 92–3.

190. Gunia S, Erbersdobler A, Hakenberg OW, Koch S, May M. p16INK4a is a marker of good prognosis for primary invasive penile squamous cell carcinoma: a multi-institutional study. J Urol. 2012; 187(3): 899–907.

191. Guimaraes GC, Leal ML, Campos RS, Zequi Sde C, da Fonseca FP, da Cunha IW, et al. Do proliferating cell nuclear antigen and MIB-1/Ki-67 have prognostic value in penile squamous cell carcinoma? Urology. 2007;70(1):137–42.

192. Guimaraes GC, de Oliveira Leal ML, Sousa Madeira Campos R, de Cassio Zequi S, da Fonseca FP, da Cunha IW, et al. Do proliferating cell nuclear antigen and MIB-1/Ki-67 have prognostic value in penile squamous cell carcinoma? Urology. 2007;70(1): 137–42.

193. Campos RS, Lopes A, Guimaraes GC, Carvalho AL, Soares FA. E-cadherin, MMP-2, and MMP-9 as prognostic markers in penile cancer: analysis of 125 patients. Urology. 2006;67(4):797–802.

194. Kroon BK, Leijte JA, van Boven H, Wessels LF, Velds A, Horenblas S, et al. Microarray gene-expression profiling to predict lymph node metastasis in penile carcinoma. BJU Int. 2008;102(4):510–5.

195. Solsona E, Iborra I, Rubio J, Casanova JL, Ricos JV, Calabuig C. Prospective validation of the association of local tumor stage and grade as a predictive factor for occult lymph node micrometastasis in patients with penile carcinoma and clinically negative inguinal lymph nodes. J Urol. 2001; 165(5):1506–9.

196. Novara G, Artibani W, Cunico SC, De Giorgi G, Gardiman M, Martignoni G, et al. How accurately do Solsona and European Association of Urology risk groups predict for risk of lymph node metastases in patients with squamous cell carcinoma of the penis? Urology. 2008;71(2): 328–33.

197. Pizzocaro G, Algaba F, Horenblas S, Solsona E, Tana S, Van Der Poel H, et al. EAU penile cancer guidelines 2009. Eur Urol. 2010;57(6):1002–12.

198. Kattan MW, Ficarra V, Artibani W, Cunico SC, Fandella A, Martignoni G, et al. Nomogram predictive of cancer specific survival in patients undergoing partial or total amputation for squamous cell carcinoma of the penis. J Urol. 2006;175(6):2103–8. discussion 8.

199. Thuret R, Sun M, Abdollah F, Schmitges J, Shariat SF, Iborra F, et al. Conditional survival predictions after surgery for patients with penile carcinoma. Cancer. 2011;117(16):3723–30.

Pathology of Penile Cancer and Its Precursor Lesions

3

Priya Rao and Pheroze Tamboli

Anatomy and Histology of the Penis

Knowledge of the anatomy and histology of the penis is essential for accurate pathologic evaluation (both gross and microscopic), pathologic tumor staging, and reporting of prognostic factors [1, 2]. The main components of the penis (glans penis, foreskin, and penile shaft) have different layers of tissue that determine the extent of invasion and therefore the pathologic stage of the tumor (Fig. 3.1). The *glans penis* has a conical shape, forming the distal end of the penis. The glans also includes the urethral meatus, the frenulum, and the corona, with the adjacent coronal sulcus forming the interface between the glans penis and the penile shaft. The anatomic layers of the glans penis from the outside in include squamous mucosa, which is usually non-keratinizing, but is keratinized in men who have been circumcised; the sub-epithelial layer or lamina propria; the corpus spongiosum, which forms most of the glans penis; and the corpora cavernosa, the length of which is variable within the glans penis. The corpora cavernosa are enclosed by the tunica albuginea, which is a thick fibroelastic sheath that acts as a barrier to invasion by tumor. The urethra is located on the ventral aspect of the glans penis, surrounded by the corpus spongiosum. Cross sections of the *penile shaft* from the outside in show skin, including dermis; dartos muscle and intermixed adipose tissue; Buck's fascia, which has loose connective tissue with numerous blood vessels and nerves; the dorsally located paired corpora cavernosa encased in the tunica albuginea, and separated by a median raphe; and the corpus spongiosum and urethra located on the ventral aspect. The *prepuce* or foreskin (from the outside in) consists of the skin, including dermis, dartos muscle, lamina propria, and squamous mucosa. The *penile root*, or bulb, is embedded in the perineum, and consists of the paired corpora cavernosa and the surrounding deep penile fascia, which is attached to the pubis by the suspensory ligament.

Arterial supply to the penis is from branches of the internal pudendal artery, which supply arterial blood to the corpus spongiosum (via the bulbar artery), the corpora cavernosa (via the cavernosal artery), and the skin, Buck's fascia, glans penis, and foreskin (via the dorsal artery). The venous drainage is via the superficial dorsal veins into the external pudendal veins, and via the deep dorsal veins into the internal pudendal veins. There is a rich network of lymphatics in the penis that drain to the superficial and deep inguinal lymph nodes, which ultimately drain into the pelvic lymph nodes.

P. Rao, M.B.B.S., M.D. • P. Tamboli, M.B.B.S. (✉)
Department of Pathology, The University of Texas
M.D. Anderson Cancer Center, 1515 Holcombe
Boulevard, Unit 85, Houston, TX 77030, USA
e-mail: ptamboli@mdanderson.org

P.E. Spiess (ed.), *Penile Cancer: Diagnosis and Treatment*, Current Clinical Urology,
DOI 10.1007/978-1-62703-367-1_3, © Springer Science+Business Media New York 2013

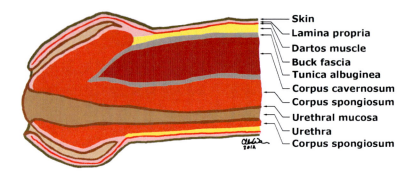

Fig. 3.1 Sagittal section of penis, showing the structures in the foreskin, penile glans, and penile shaft. Figure courtesy of Chloe A. Walker

Premalignant Lesions of the Penis

Premalignant lesions involving the penis have been referred to in various ways in the pathology literature including low- and high-grade squamous intraepithelial lesion; mild, moderate, and severe dysplasia; dysplasia and carcinoma in situ; and penile intraepithelial neoplasia (PeIN) [3–6]. Erythroplasia of Queyrat, Bowen's disease, and Bowenoid papulosis are the clinical terms used when the lesion has histologic features of squamous cell carcinoma (SCC) in situ. However, Bowenoid papulosis is not a true premalignant lesion. Lichen sclerosus, while not a true premalignant lesion, is also discussed in this section because of its association with a subset of SCCs of the penis.

PeIN is the nomenclature proposed by Cubilla et al., for pre-neoplastic squamous lesions affecting the penis [6, 7]. They have divided PeIN into differentiated and undifferentiated, with rare cases of mixed differentiated and undifferentiated PeIN. Cubilla's group has also reported correlation between the type of PeIN and the accompanying invasive SCC [8]. *Differentiated PeIN* is considered to be the premalignant lesion for well-differentiated and -keratinized SCC, and is associated with lichen sclerosus. Differentiated PeIN is not related to human papilloma virus (HPV) infection, affects older men, and most commonly involves the foreskin, and the glans penis less frequently, forming a macule or irregular plaque. Microscopically, these are flat lesions

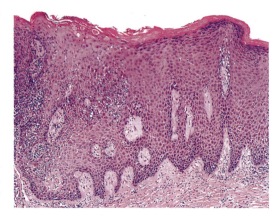

Fig. 3.2 Penile intraepithelial neoplasia (PeIN), differentiated type. H&E, 100×

resembling typical well-differentiated squamous carcinoma with low nuclear grade and variable degrees of keratinization (Fig. 3.2). These lesions are morphologically equivalent to mild and moderate squamous dysplasia, and may be found adjacent to invasive squamous carcinoma. Immunohistochemical stain for p53 is usually positive in these lesions, while p16 stain is negative. Ki-67 usually stains the lower third of cells in these lesions. *Undifferentiated PeIN* is equivalent to SCC in situ, with close to 90% of lesions associated with HPV infection [8–10]. These lesions generally affect the glans penis, and are considered to be the premalignant precursors of HPV-related SCC, such as basaloid and warty SCC. Microscopically, undifferentiated PeIN may show basaloid, warty, or mixed features. Basaloid PeIN has morphologic features similar

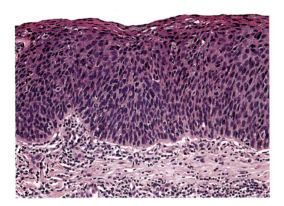

Fig. 3.3 Penile intraepithelial neoplasia (PeIN), undifferentiated type with basaloid features. The neoplastic cells have morphologic features similar to those seen in basaloid squamous cell carcinoma (see Fig. 3.21). H&E, 200×

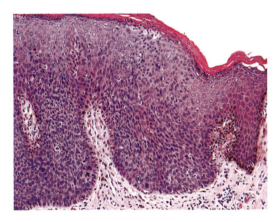

Fig. 3.4 Penile intraepithelial neoplasia (PeIN), undifferentiated type with basaloid features. The neoplastic cells are compared to the normal hyperplastic cells (present on the *right*). H&E, 150×

to basaloid SCC, with small- to intermediate-sized cells that have a high nucleus-to-cytoplasmic ratio, frequent mitoses, and apoptosis (Figs. 3.3 and 3.4). Immunohistochemical stain for p16 is reported to be positive in most basaloid PeIN. Warty PeIN, as the name suggests, has prominent pleomorphic koilocytic features similar to those seen in warty (condylomatous) SCC. Some lesions may have a mixture of warty and basaloid features and are referred to as mixed.

Erythroplasia of Queyrat, Bowen's disease, and Bowenoid papulosis have a similar histologic appearance, but different clinical presentation and biologic behavior. *Erythroplasia of Queyrat* usually affects men in the fourth and fifth decades of life, but has also been reported in younger and older men. Clinically, the lesion forms an elevated, moist-appearing, erythematous plaque, which is usually located on the glans penis or sometimes on the mucosal (inner) aspect of the foreskin [11]. Most lesions are solitary; however, there may be multiple lesions. Microscopically, it looks like typical SCC in situ seen elsewhere, but usually with a band-like lymphocytic infiltrate in the underlying stroma. Clinically, the differential diagnosis includes Zoon's balanitis, psoriasis, drug eruption, and inflammatory processes; however, pathologic diagnosis is straightforward. Invasive SCC develops in approximately 10% of patients [11].

Bowen's disease is the term used to designate SCC in situ that occurs on the shaft, and is not erythematous like erythroplasia of Queyrat [12, 13]. Peak incidence is in the fifth and sixth decades of life. Clinically, these lesions form crusted, sharply demarcated, scaly white plaques on the penile skin. Microscopically, they are typical of SCC in situ [11, 13]. Approximately 5–10% of cases are reported to progress to invasive SCC. Two studies, one from 1973 [11] and the other from 1980 [14], reported that a number of patients also developed other cutaneous and/or extra-cutaneous malignancies. However, these findings have not been confirmed in more recent literature.

Bowenoid papulosis is the term used for multicentric SCC in situ associated with HPV [15, 16]. HPV types 16 and 18 are the ones most commonly associated with these lesions [17]. This condition usually affects young men, and is regarded as the male counterpart of the multifocal vulvo-vaginal dysplasia seen in young women. Clinically, there are multiple small (2–10 mm) soft papules mostly on the penile shaft, and occasionally on the glans or the foreskin. The papules may coalesce to form plaques, which resemble condyloma acuminata. Microscopically, these lesions show typical histological features of SCC in situ. For this reason the diagnosis of Bowenoid papulosis is not rendered on microscopic features

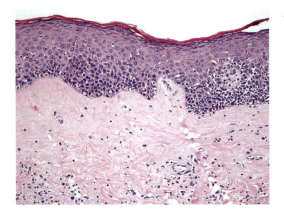

Fig. 3.5 Lichen sclerosus, showing flattened squamous epithelium, inflammatory cells, and a hyalinized stroma. H&E, 100×

alone; rather, the clinical presentation and gross appearance need to be taken into account before making this diagnosis. The natural history of this lesion differs significantly from that of Bowen's disease and erythroplasia of Queryat, as Bowenoid papulosis does not progress to invasive SCC, has an indolent clinical course, and may undergo spontaneous regression. These lesions are treated conservatively by local excision, and topical or laser treatment.

Lichen sclerosus, although not a true premalignant lesion, is briefly discussed here as it is associated with a subset of SCC that are not related to HPV infection, and also with some variants, such as papillary NOS, verrucous, and pseudohyperplastic SCC [18]. Lichen sclerosus is a chronic inflammatory disorder with stromal sclerosis and epithelial atrophy, which affects the penis and vulva. While the term balanitis xerotica obliterans has been used interchangeably for this lesion, lichen sclerosus is the preferred term. This lesion affects the mucosal surface of the foreskin and the glans penis, forming atrophic appearing irregular gray-white areas. Eventually, these lesions form a smooth surface due to the underlying stromal sclerosis, as opposed to the normal wrinkled surface of the foreskin and glans. Morphologically, the squamous epithelium is flattened due to loss of rete ridges, there is a lichenoid inflammatory infiltrate below the epithelium and also in the epithelium, and eventually there is hyalinization of the sub-epithelial stroma (Fig. 3.5).

Squamous Cell Carcinoma of the Penis

SCC is the most common malignant tumor affecting the penis. SCCs of the penis tend to affect older men, with a mean age at presentation of 58 years, as reported in the literature [19–22]. These tumors are rare in men under the age of 40 years, but have been reported in all age groups, including children, and even men in their ninth decade. Most patients present with a penile mass, which may be exophytic or ulcerated. Penile pain, urethral discharge, difficulty in urination, bleeding from the penis or urethra, and inguinal lymphadenopathy due to metastases may also be present at the time of initial diagnosis. These tumors exhibit a variety of morphologic patterns, some of which are of prognostic significance.

Majority of SCCs arise from the glans penis, with fewer tumors affecting the foreskin, coronal sulcus, and penile shaft. The tumor's *site of origin* affects what layers of the penis are invaded by tumor and therefore impact the pathologic stage. Tumors involving the foreskin have the best outcome, as these generally do not invade into the corpus spongiosum or corpora cavernosa of the glans or the shaft. Of course, larger tumors may involve more than one anatomic structure, making it difficult to ascertain the exact site of origin [19, 20, 22]. Moreover, SCC may grow as multifocal tumors, with two or more independent foci of carcinoma separated by benign tissue. These tumors tend to be superficial, and the foci of tumor are separated by benign-appearing squamous epithelium, which may be either normal or hyperplastic.

Patterns of Growth of Penile Squamous Cell Carcinoma

SCCs tend to have a variety of different growth patterns (verruciform, superficial spreading, vertical), some of which are of prognostic importance [23–25]. Tumors with a *verruciform growth pattern* mostly involve the glans penis, and are exophytic, with a papillary or cauliflower-like external surface and a well-defined tumor base [12]. Microscopically, these tend to be low-grade tumors that show one of the three distinctive morphologic types, i.e., verrucous, warty (condylomatous), and papillary not otherwise specified (NOS). Most of these tumors invade only into the lamina propria, and rarely invade into the corpus spongiosum of the glans penis [26]. *Superficial spreading* SCCs tend to grow slowly and horizontally along the mucosal surface of the glans, coronal sulcus, or foreskin, potentially involving more than one site, as they tend to cover a wide surface area. SCCs with this pattern of growth form an elevated, firm plaque-like or band-like mass, the surface of which may be granular or ulcerated. Microscopically, most of the tumor is in situ, well to moderately differentiated, with few foci of invasion into the superficial lamina propria. Rare tumors may progress to a vertical growth phase with invasion into deeper layers. SCCs that grow with a superficial spreading pattern rarely metastasize, and have a favorable prognosis. Awareness of this pattern of growth is important for urologists, as these tumors may occupy a larger area than antici-pated. Achieving negative surgical margins, especially in partial penectomy specimens, is of concern with this growth pattern [27]. Tumors with a *vertical growth pattern* invade vertically down, usually into the corpus spongiosum or through the tunica albuginea deep into the corpora cavernosa, surrounding the urethra or sometimes replacing it [12]. Grossly, they typically form large, fungating, and often ulcerated masses. Hemorrhage and necrosis are common. Satellite tumor nodules may be present, often located deep in the corpora cavernosa. These are often high-grade tumors with the worst prognosis, and a high rate of inguinal lymph node metastasis. A *mixed growth pattern* may be composed of superficial spreading, verruciform, or vertical growth components, in varying proportions. Microscopically, there may be a combination of low- and high-grade tumor histology.

Morphologic Types of Penile Squamous Cell Carcinoma

Morphologically, penile carcinomas may be divided into SCC of usual type (70%), verruci-form carcinomas (25%, including papillary

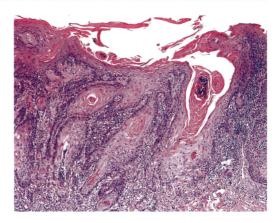

Fig. 3.6 Squamous cell carcinoma (usual type) invading into the underlying lamina propria. H&E, 40×

carcinoma NOS, warty carcinoma, and verrucous carcinoma), basaloid carcinoma, mixed carcinomas, and sarcomatoid carcinoma. Histologic types, other than the usual type, have distinct morphologic features involving the majority of the tumor, which is arbitrarily defined as more than 80% of the sampled tumor. SCC (usual type) may occa-sionally exhibit small foci of the other patterns. Each of these histologic types is discussed indi-vidually in the subsequent sections.

Squamous Cell Carcinoma (Usual Type)

SCC (usual type) is morphologically similar to SCC occurring in the skin or other organs (Figs. 3.6, 3.7, 3.8, 3.9, and 3.10) [25, 28]. Tumor cells are arranged in nests or cords with variable amounts of keratinization, depending on the degree of differ-entiation (Fig. 3.7). The majority of these tumors are moderately differentiated, with the remaining smaller subset being either well or poorly differen-tiated (Fig. 3.8). High-grade tumors may have a pseudoglandular appearance, secondary to acan-tholysis, with the gland-like spaces lined by flattened squamous cells. These spaces may be empty or contain keratin or inflammatory and necrotic debris (Fig. 3.9). Small foci of spindle cells may also be present in some poorly differenti-ated SCC, but these need to be differentiated from sarcomatoid dedifferentiation. The stroma around the tumor cells is reactive and may have varying amounts of inflammatory infiltrate. Most of these tumors are straightforward to diagnose as they are accompanied by adjacent carcinoma in situ.

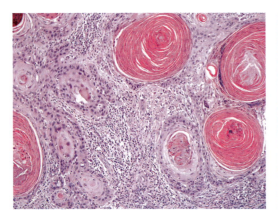

Fig. 3.7 Squamous cell carcinoma (usual type), well differentiated. Intermediate power view showing *pink whorls* of keratin in the tumor nests. H&E, 100×

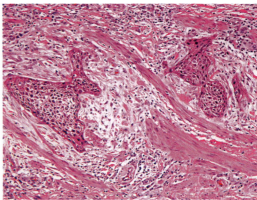

Fig. 3.10 Squamous cell carcinoma (usual type), invading into the dartos muscle in the foreskin. H&E, 100×

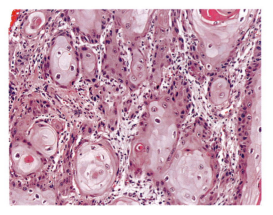

Fig. 3.8 Squamous cell carcinoma (usual type), moderately differentiated. Intermediate power view showing tumor cells with eosinophilic (*pink*) glassy cytoplasm. H&E, 200×

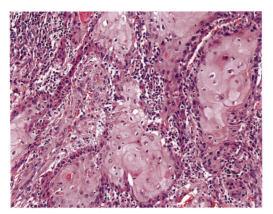

Fig. 3.9 Squamous cell carcinoma (usual type), moderately differentiated. Intermediate power view showing tumor nests surrounded by inflammatory cells. H&E, 200×

In some cases, these tumors need to be differentiated from pseudoepitheliomatous hyperplasia, metastasis of SCC to the penis, and extension of carcinoma from the urethra. Occasionally, poorly differentiated usual type SCC may be difficult to differentiate from basaloid SCC; a differential diagnosis that may be resolved by HPV testing as all basaloid SCCs are positive for HPV, while usual type SCCs are negative. The distinction from poorly differentiated carcinoma of the urethra is important for therapeutic purposes; especially for urethral tumors extending from the urethral meatus with focal involvement of the adjacent glans penis. Urethral tumors may be managed by excision of the urethra, while penile tumors generally require a partial or total penectomy, depending on the extent of the tumor. Urethral carcinomas generally show carcinoma in situ along the penile urethra, which is rare in penile tumors.

Locoregional recurrences have been reported in up to 28% of patients, usually secondary to inadequate surgical resection [28]. Metastases to the inguinal lymph nodes have been reported to range from 28 to 39% [25, 28]. A 10-year survival rate of 78% has been reported in one series, with mortality rates reported to vary from 20 to 38% [25, 28].

Papillary Carcinoma, Not Otherwise Specified

Papillary carcinoma NOS is the most common type of SCC with a verruciform growth pattern, ranging from 5 to 15% of all penile SCCs [25, 28]. These tumors most commonly arise on the glans and foreskin, and rarely in the coronal sulcus. They form a cauliflower-like, firm, gray-white mass. On cut section, the tumor surface appears serrated, and the papillae are visible as white fingerlike projections, which are the areas of keratinization that are best seen after formalin fixation. The interface between tumor and the underlying stroma is poorly demarcated. Grossly visible invasion into the underlying tissue, including the dartos muscle and corpus spongiosum, is common.

Microscopically, these tumors are mainly composed of variable length papillae lined by malignant cells with acanthosis and hyperkeratosis (Figs. 3.11, 3.12, and 3.13). The tumor cells lack the condylomatous features seen in condyloma accuminatum and warty (condylomatous) carcinoma. These carcinomas have an irregular infiltrative border, with jagged irregular nests of tumor cells invading the underlying stroma (Fig. 3.13); however, they rarely invade into corpora cavernosa. Lymphovascular and perineural invasion are not commonly present in these tumors. The most common differential diagnostic entities to be ruled out include warty (condylomaotus) carcinoma and verrucous carcinoma. Moreover, the diagnosis of this tumor can only be rendered after unequivocal exclusion of both warty (condylomatous) SCC and verrucous SCC. Warty (condylomatous) carcinomas have distinctive HPV-related changes and tend to show a higher degree of nuclear pleomorphism. Further, unlike warty (condylomatous) SCC, papillary NOS SCCs are negative for HPV and p16 [10]. Verrucous carcinomas have the characteristic bulbous smooth pushing border, compared to the jagged and irregular one present in most papillary carcinomas, and minimal to no cytologic atypia.

Locoregional recurrences have been reported in up to 12% of patients, and the rate of inguinal lymph node metastases has been reported to be from 0 to 12% [25, 28]. In the series from Cubilla et al., patients with these tumors had a 90% 5-year survival rate [12, 29]. The reported mortality rate is low, varying from 0 to 6% [25, 28].

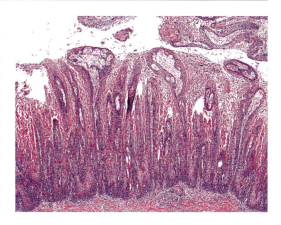

Fig. 3.11 Papillary NOS squamous cell carcinoma. Low-power view shows the papillary architecture of the tumor. H&E, 20×

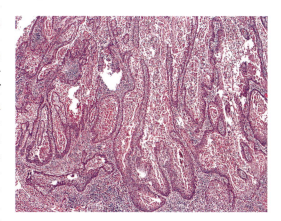

Fig. 3.12 Papillary NOS squamous cell carcinoma. Low-power view showing the papillary architecture of the tumor, with keratin and cellular debris in between the papillary fronds. H&E, 40×

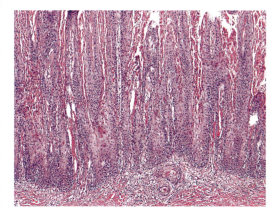

Fig. 3.13 Papillary NOS squamous cell carcinoma. Low-power view showing the papillary architecture of the tumor, with a small nest infiltrating into the lamina propria (just to the *right of center*). H&E, 40×

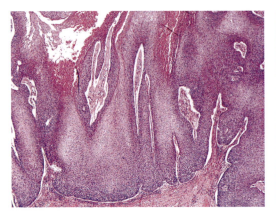

Fig. 3.14 Warty (condylomatous) squamous cell carcinoma. Low-power view showing a verruciform tumor pushing into the underlying stroma. H&E, 20×

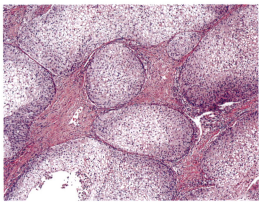

Fig. 3.15 Warty (condylomatous) squamous cell carcinoma. Low-power view shows large nest of tumor cells invading into the lamina propria. H&E, 40×

Warty (Condylomatous) Carcinoma

Warty (condylomatous) carcinoma is related to HPV infection, and is reported to be 6–10% of all penile SCCs [28, 30]. Clinically, these tumors tend to grow slowly; however, a small percentage of patients may present with metastases to the inguinal lymph nodes. Interestingly, these tumors tend to affect younger men, who are usually about 10 years younger than the average patient with usual type SCC. These carcinomas also form cauliflower-like, firm, gray-white growths, which may be quite large (average 4 cm reported by Cubilla et al.). These usually grow on the glans penis, but may be multicentric [26]. On cut section, the tumor has distinct exophytic and endophytic components, with a well-demarcated interface between the tumor and underlying tissue, which is the lamina propria and corpus spongiosum in most cases. The corpora cavernosa are rarely invaded.

Microscopically, the tumor is composed of long papillae lined by tumor cells with prominent koilocytic atypia, similar to that present in other HPV-related lesions (Figs. 3.14, 3.15, 3.16, and 3.17). The tumor surface shows prominent hyperkeratosis and atypical parakeratosis, leading to the gray-white gross appearance. The tumor nuclei are large, wrinkled, and hyperchromatic, and cells may be binucleated or even multinucleated. Numerous mitoses and apoptotic bodies are present. The prominent koilocytic atypia is typical of this SCC (Figs. 3.16 and 3.17),

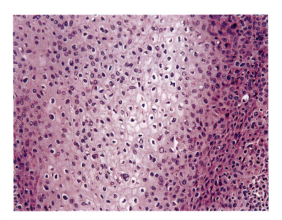

Fig. 3.16 Warty (condylomatous) squamous cell carcinoma. High-power view shows tumor cells with koilocytic features. H&E, 200×

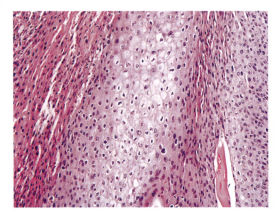

Fig. 3.17 Warty (condylomatous) squamous cell carcinoma. High-power view shows tumor cells with koilocytic features. H&E, 200×

and is not seen in the other squamous carcinomas with a verruciform growth pattern (papillary NOS and verrucous carcinoma). Up to one-third of these carcinomas may be associated with a benign condyloma. Identification of HPV in warty SCC has been variably reported, ranging from 22 to 100%. This wide discrepancy is probably related to the use of different techniques for HPV detection [31]. In contrast to HPV, p16 is consistently positive in warty SCC.

The *giant condyloma of Buschke–Lowenstein* is the most important differential diagnostic consideration in this type of SCC, especially when there is limited or superficial sampling of the penile tumor. Giant condylomas have HPV-induced koilocytic features similar to warty carcinoma, but lack the nuclear pleomorphism seen in warty SCC. Giant condylomas generally also have a bulbous expansion at the base that pushes into the underlying stroma, somewhat similar to that seen in verrucous carcinoma, unlike the irregular nests of invasion in warty SCC. In contrast, the nuclear atypia in warty carcinomas is malignant appearing, and most important there is destructive stromal invasion with jagged nests of tumor cells invading the underlying tissue. Verrucous carcinomas lack the condylomatous features, papillae, and koilocytic atypia and have a broad-based pushing interface with the underlying tissue. Papillary NOS SCCs have the most overlapping morphologic features with warty SCC, including condylomatous features, papillae, and irregular nests. However, papillary NOS SCCs lack the koilocytic atypia and HPV that are present in warty SCC. Finally, some cases of usual type SCC have cells with clear cytoplasm that mimic koilocytic cells, but lack the nuclear features, papillary architecture, and condylomatous features of warty SCC.

Locoregional recurrences have been reported in up to 10% of patients, and about 18% of patients have metastases to the inguinal lymph nodes [25, 26, 28]. As with papillary NOS SCC, these tumors are less aggressive, with a 90% 5-year survival as reported by Cubilla and colleagues [26]. The reported mortality rate is similarly low, ranging from 0 to 9% [25, 28].

Verrucous Carcinoma

Verrucous carcinoma of the penis is a well-differentiated neoplasm, which in some series accounts for 3–7% of all penile cancers [25, 28]. The lack of consistent use of morphologic criteria for rendering this diagnosis makes it difficult to ascertain its true incidence, especially when perusing the older scientific literature [12, 32–35].

Similar to the other verruciform tumors (papillary carcinoma NOS and warty carcinoma), verrucous carcinomas tend to grow slowly, forming an exophytic, cauliflower-like white to gray firm tumor, the surface of which may be ulcerated. Also like the other verruciform tumors, this carcinoma involves the glans penis most commonly, occasionally involving the foreskin. These tumors usually present as a single tumor, but may be multicentric. The cut surface of the tumor shows the exophytic component with a sharply demarcated interface with the underlying tissue. An endophytic component may be present consisting of broad-based nests pushing into the stroma.

Microscopically, verrucous carcinoma is well differentiated with the exophytic component showing prominent papillomatosis, hyperkeratosis, parakeratosis, and acanthosis (Figs. 3.18 and 3.19). In contrast to papillary carcinoma NOS, the papillae in verrucous carcinoma usually lack a central fibrovascular core. A characteristic feature of this carcinoma is the endophytic component, which consists of broad-based bulbous projections at the base of the tumor that may push deeply into the lamina propria forming a regular pushing border. A dense inflammatory infiltrate may be present at the interface of the tumor and penile stroma, which may occasionally obscure the interface. These bulbous projections are in contrast to the irregular jagged nests characteristic of the invasion present in other forms of invasive SCC. Tumor cells have prominent intercellular bridges, and show no or minimal nuclear atypia. Some cells with vacuolated cytoplasm may be seen on the surface; however, these are quite distinct from koilocytic cells. Rare mitoses may be seen at the base of the bulbous nests. Verrucous carcinomas are negative for HPV [10]; however, in the older literature, one may find cases reported as positive,

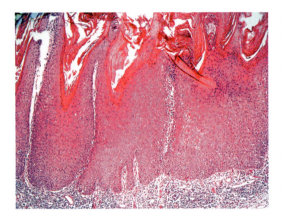

Fig. 3.18 Verrucous carcinoma of the penis, showing an exophytic growth at the *top* and large bulbous nests of tumor cells pushing into the underlying stroma at the *bottom*. H&E, 40×

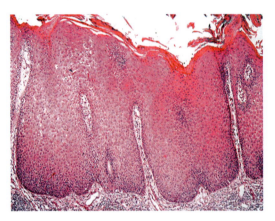

Fig. 3.19 Verrucous carcinoma of the penis, showing large bulbous nests of tumor cells pushing into the underlying stroma. H&E, 40×

which probably represent tumors that today would not be classified as verrucous carcinoma.

Some tumors may be predominantly verrucous with a variable amount (sometimes focal) of other types of SCC. The other squamous cell carcinoma components may form invasive irregular jagged nests of atypical malignant cells, in contrast to the bulbous nests of verrucous carcinoma. Some of these tumors with mixed morphologic features of verrucous carcinoma and other SCC types are more appropriately designated as mixed SCC. This is important to note, as pure verrucous carcinomas, i.e., those without other types of SCC, do not metastasize to the lymph nodes. However, local recurrences may occur if surgical excision is not adequate and the margins of resection are positive for tumor.

Giant condyloma of Buschke–Lowenstein, warty carcinoma, and papillary carcinoma NOS are the important considerations in the differential diagnosis of verrucous carcinoma. Giant condylomas of Buschke–Lowenstein and warty carcinoma have characteristic HPV-related koilocytic changes that are not present in verrucous carcinoma. Warty carcinomas also have a greater degree of cytologic atypia and irregular nests of invasive tumor, as opposed to the broad-based tumor nests in verrucous carcinoma. Papillary carcinoma NOS exhibits papillae with a central fibrovascular core, has a greater degree of cytologic atypia, and has irregular nests of invasive tumor at the base.

Pure verrucous carcinomas recur locally if the primary excision is inadequate; however, the local recurrence may constitute a higher grade SCC without verrucous features. Most importantly, these tumors never metastasize to the inguinal lymph nodes, which makes inguinal lymph node dissection unnecessary in cases of pure verrucous carcinoma (i.e., tumors without other admixed SCC types) [25, 28, 36]. In recent studies, no patients with pure verrucous carcinoma have been reported to die of disease [25, 28].

Basaloid Carcinoma

Basaloid carcinoma of the penis is a highly malignant HPV-related carcinoma, which is fast growing and deeply invasive. This type of SCC accounts for 10–14% of all penile SCC. As with warty SCC, another HPV-related SCC, basaloid SCC occurs in younger patients than those with usual type SCC. Basaloid SCCs have a poor prognosis with a high rate of local recurrence and lymph node metastasis. In one series, two-thirds of all patients with basaloid carcinoma had inguinal lymph node metastases at initial presentation [37].

Basaloid SCCs are generally large, with an average tumor size >4 cm reported in the series from Cubilla et al. [37]. These tumors are usually located on the glans penis, forming irregular, gray to red tumors most often with surface ulceration. The tumor may also involve the adjacent coronal sulcus and foreskin, and less frequently

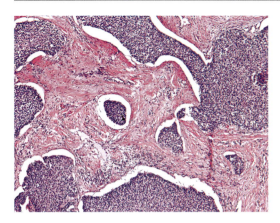

Fig. 3.20 Basaloid squamous cell carcinoma, showing nests of small dark cells, infiltrating the corpus spongiosum. H&E, 40×

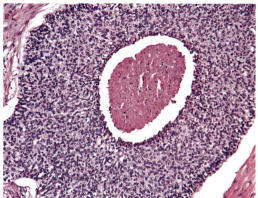

Fig. 3.22 Basaloid squamous cell carcinoma, with comedo necrosis in a large nest of tumor with uniform cells with *dark* nuclei. H&E, 100×

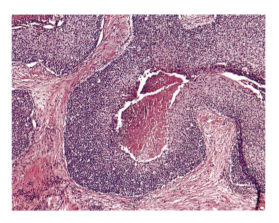

Fig. 3.21 Basaloid squamous cell carcinoma, with comedo necrosis in a large nest of tumor with *dark* cells and foci of apoptosis leading to a "starry sky"-like appearance. H&E, 40×

the skin of the penile shaft. On cut section, the tumor has a deeply invasive vertical growth pattern, with a rounded or slightly lobulated contour, and multiple minute foci of tumor necrosis.

Microscopically, this carcinoma is characteristically composed of solid nests of small, poorly differentiated basaloid cells, with numerous foci of central comedo necrosis (Figs. 3.20, 3.21, and 3.22). The tumor cells are small, uniform, with basophilic cytoplasm and dark nuclei with inconspicuous nucleoli. Spindled cells may be present, but these also have a basaloid appearance. Mitoses are numerous, and the abundant apoptotic cells

create a "starry sky" appearance (Fig. 3.21). Keratinization may be focally present, usually in the center of the nests, along with comedo necrosis. Perineural invasion and lymphovascular invasion are frequent, leading to the high rate of lymph node metastases. These carcinomas tend to be deeply invasive, with frequent extension into the corpora cavernosa. HPV is usually positive in basaloid SCC, with HPV-16 serotype being the most common. p16 immunohistochemical stain is consistently positive in these tumors.

The differential diagnosis includes poorly differentiated urethral carcinoma and basal cell carcinoma. Urethral carcinomas exhibit a greater degree of nuclear pleomorphism, and usually have an associated papillary component or carcinoma in situ along the urethral mucosa. Basal cell carcinoma is rare, and typically involves the skin of the shaft; in contrast basaloid SCC affects the glans penis. Nests of basal cell carcinoma show nuclear palisading, and lack the high mitotic rate, apoptotic cells, and comedo necrosis present in basaloid SCC.

High rates (up to 36%) of local recurrences have been reported in patients treated with a partial penectomy [28, 38]. A large number of patients are reported to have metastases to the inguinal lymph nodes, ranging from 50 to 100% [25, 28, 36, 37]. These tumors are highly aggressive, with a 76% 10-year survival rate reported by Guimaraes and colleagues [28]. The reported mortality rate ranges from 27 to 67% [25, 28, 37].

Squamous Cell Carcinoma with Sarcomatoid Dedifferentiation

SCCs with sarcomatoid dedifferentiation, similar to other carcinomas in the genitourinary tract with sarcomatoid dedifferentiation, are rare but aggressive tumors that are predominantly composed of spindle cells [39, 40]. Grossly, they form bulky, gray-white or -red, fungating or polypoid masses, and most commonly involve the glans penis. Like the basaloid SCC, they have a vertical pattern of growth, being deeply invasive into corpus spongiosum and corpora cavernosa. Smaller satellite tumor nodules may also be present, sometimes in the corpora cavernosa or in the skin of the penis. The tumor has a biphasic appearance (sarcomatoid and epithelial) as with other carcinomas with sarcomatoid dedifferentiation. The malignant spindle cell (sarcomatoid) component may be prominent, usually forming fascicles that resemble either fibrosarcoma or leiomyosarcoma. The sarcomatoid component may resemble malignant fibrous histiocytoma (MFH), with giant cells and pleomorphic epithelioid cells. Rare tumors may have a sarcomatoid component mimicking angiosarcoma. Necrosis and mitoses are usually prominent. In some cases, the epithelial SCC component may be minimal or absent. In the absence of the epithelial SCC, a prior history of SCC, and/or the presence of squamous dysplasia or squamous carcinoma in situ in the adjacent mucosa, helps establish the diagnosis. Cytokeratin and epithelial membrane antigen (EMA) immunohistochemical stains may help confirm the epithelial origin of the spindle cells of the sarcomatoid component; however, these stains are not always positive in the spindle cell component. High-molecular-weight cytokeratin (34βE12), p63, and vimentin immunohistochemical stains have also been reported to be positive in the sarcomatoid component [39]. Primary sarcomas of the penis (leiomyosarcoma most often) and spindle cell melanoma are the most common differential diagnostic considerations, which can most often be excluded by the use of immunohistochemical stains.

SCCs with sarcomatoid dedifferentiation are aggressive tumors, which may present with lymph node and visceral metastases. Metastases to the inguinal lymph nodes have been reported in 75–89% of patients [39, 40]. The mortality rate is reported to range from 40 to 75% [39, 40].

Other Squamous Carcinoma Types

Rare types of squamous carcinoma include mixed carcinoma, warty–basaloid carcinoma, adenosquamous carcinoma, pseudohyperplastic carcinoma, pseudoglandular carcinoma, and carcinoma cuniculatum.

Mixed carcinomas exhibit two or more different histologic types of SCC. The most common mixed carcinoma is a typical verrucous carcinoma with foci of moderately or poorly differentiated SCC. These tumors have been referred to as hybrid carcinomas by some authors [12, 41]. Mixed carcinomas composed of usual type SCC, basaloid carcinoma, or other types are seen rarely. Combinations of basaloid carcinoma and warty carcinoma, both HPV-related carcinomas, have also been reported. A few mixed carcinomas have been reported to show no significant differences in outcome compared to verrucous carcinoma after similar treatment.

Warty–basaloid carcinomas are HPV-related mixed carcinomas that have features of both warty and basaloid SCC. A case series of 45 patients was recently reported by Chaux et al. [42]. Two-thirds of their cases had the typical morphologic features of warty SCC on the surface and features of basaloid SCC in the deeply infiltrative nests. In a smaller number of tumors, the nests of invasive carcinoma had mixed morphologic features of basaloid and warty SCC. Most tumors were invasive into corpus spongiosum and/or corpora cavernosa. Lymphovascular invasion and perineural invasion were common, similar to basaloid SCC, leading to metastases to inguinal lymph nodes. The clinical significance of these tumors lies in their biologic behavior, which is similar to that of basaloid SCC rather than warty SCC.

Adenosquamous carcinomas are rare tumors composed of SCC with a mixture of glandular elements that may have luminal mucin expression [43]. SCCs with acantholysis need to be considered in the differential diagnosis [43].

Pseudohyperplastic SCC is a well-differentiated carcinoma that usually involves the foreskin and is associated with lichen sclerosus. This tumor is morphologically characterized by nests of keratinizing squamous cells with minimal atypia, which are set within a reactive stroma. This type of SCC may be confused with pseudoepitheliomatous hyperplasia, especially in limited tissue biopsy samples [44].

Pseudoglandular SCC is a rare variant with prominent acantholysis leading to the formation of pseudoglandular spaces [45].

Carcinoma cuniculatum is a well-differentiated SCC that has a tendency to burrow deeply, often forming fistula-like tracts [46].

Pathology Reporting and Predictive Pathology Features in Penile Squamous Cell Carcinoma

Pathology plays a critical role in the accurate diagnosis and staging of penile SCC. A thorough detailed gross assessment which includes tumor size, location, and extent of penile involvement is the first step toward accurate pathologic staging. Also, certain histologic features are known to be predictive of patient outcome. The salient predictive histologic parameters that are reported to be of clinical significance are discussed below. More detailed information regarding prognosis is discussed in Chap. 2.

Pathologic Reporting of Penile Squamous Cell Carcinoma

The Cancer Committee of the College of American Pathologists (CAP) has developed tumor-specific checklists called Cancer Protocols, for pathologists to use when reporting cancer diagnoses. These checklists contain scientifically validated data elements that must be reported in all tumor types, for which a cancer protocol exists, in order to maintain pathology laboratory accreditation. Since 2004, the American College of Surgeons' Commission on Cancer program accreditation has also mandated that at least 90%

Table 3.1 Pathologic reporting of penile squamous cell carcinoma

Type of specimen (penectomy partial vs. total, circumcision, other)
Tumor site
Tumor size
Histologic subtype
Histologic grade (well, moderate, or poor)
Depth of invasion (lamina propria, corpus spongiosum, dartos, corpora cavernosa)
Lymphovascular or perineural invasion
Surgical resection margins
Pathologic TNM stage

of all pathology reports from cancer specimens include all required data elements from these CAP Cancer Protocols. In addition, in 2009, the Canadian Association of Pathologists unanimously endorsed the adoption of the CAP Cancer Protocols. These protocols are updated periodically as new data becomes readily available, and the current version of the protocol for penile SCC was last updated in 2011 (http://www.cap.org). The key pathologic features that must be included in all pathology reports for penile tumor specimens are summarized in Table 3.1.

Histologic Subtype of Primary Tumor

The histologic subtypes of penile SCC have been discussed in detail above in Sect. "Morphologic Types of Penile Squamous Cell Carcinoma." The subtype of penile SCC should be specified in the pathology report, as the different subtypes have distinctly different prognostic and therapeutic implications. As discussed in the above-mentioned section basaloid SCC, mixed basaloid and warty SCC, SCC with sarcomatoid dedifferentiation, and adenosquamous carcinoma are associated with the worst outcomes [25, 28]. Conversely, warty SCC, verrucous SCC, and papillary NOS subtypes have better prognosis, with warty and papillary NOS having a relatively low rate of regional lymph node metastasis. Pure verrucous SCCs do not metastasize and generally do not require an inguinal lymph node dissection.

Tumor Grade

Tumor grade is a strong independent prognosticator of lymph node metastasis. SCC of the penis is typically stratified into three grades of differentiation (well, moderate, and poor) depending on the amount of cellular differentiation displayed by the tumor cells and the percentage of each component. A recently proposed three-tier grading system also divides tumors based on the degree of differentiation into the following: grade 1 tumor cells are well differentiated, with tumor cells that are morphologically similar to normal squamous cells with minimal nuclear atypia; grade 2 tumors have cells with eosinophilic keratinized-appearing cytoplasm, minimal to moderate nuclear pleomorphism, and visible or prominent nucleoli; finally, grade 3 tumors have anaplastic cells without the distinctive squamous appearance, pleomorphic nuclei, prominent nucleoli, and multiple mitoses (Fig. 3.23) [47, 48]. These authors argue that any proportion of grade 3 tumor cells have a higher rate of nodal metastases compared to tumors without any grade 3 component [48]. This view differs from that reported by Slaton et al. (albeit it is not so significantly different) who reported that tumors which display greater than 50% poorly differentiated (grade 3) foci were associated with a much higher percentage (60%) of regional lymph node metastasis, when compared with tumors with less than 50% poorly differentiated (grade 3) component that exhibit only a 15% likelihood of nodal metastases [49].

Extent of Invasion and TNM Pathologic Stage

There is excellent correlation between the TNM pathologic stage of penile carcinomas and the occurrence of lymph node metastasis [49, 50]. As with all other tumors the higher the pathologic stage the worse the biologic behavior. The pathologic tumor stage (pT) is based on the depth of invasion, i.e., what anatomic structures are directly invaded by the tumor (see Table 3.2). pT1 tumors have been found to have a low risk of lymphovascular invasion and/or regional lymph

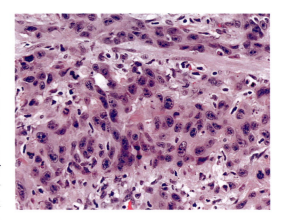

Fig. 3.23 Squamous cell carcinoma (usual type), poorly differentiated. High-power view showing tumor cells with grade 3 features. H&E, 200×

node metastasis. Conversely, over half of the pT2 tumors are also associated with both lymphovascular invasion and lymph node metastasis [49]. In 2008, Leijte et al. proposed a modification of the current staging scheme for penile tumors. They found that tumors that invade the corpus cavernosum have an adverse prognosis in comparison to tumors that are confined to the corpus spongiosum [51]. The authors proposed modifying the current staging scheme to include tumors with corpus cavernosum involvement in the pT3 category, thus stratifying patients based upon prognostic outcomes [51]. However, this proposed change was not included in the 2010 TNM classification, which is outlined in Table 3.2.

Correlation between the depth of invasion, as measured in millimeters, and outcome has also been reported [1, 47]. However, this prognostic factor has not gained widespread acceptance.

Lymphovascular Invasion

Lymphovascular invasion is an independent prognostic factor and is predictive of lymph node metastasis [49, 52, 53]. The presence of tumor in lymphovascular spaces (Fig. 3.24) is associated with reduced 5-year survival rates [53]. The presence or the absence of lymphovascular invasion is a pertinent histologic parameter that must be included in all pathologic reports.

Table 3.2 Tumor node metastasis (TNM) staging of penile squamous cell carcinoma

pT: Primary tumor stage	
pTX	Primary tumor cannot be assessed
pT0	No evidence of primary tumor
pTis	Carcinoma in situ
pTa	Noninvasive verrucous carcinoma
pT1a	Tumor invades sub-epithelial connective tissue without lymphovascular invasion and is not poorly differentiated (i.e., grade 3–4)
pT1b	Tumor invades sub-epithelial connective tissue with lymphovascular invasion or is poorly differentiated
pT2	Tumor invades corpus spongiosum or cavernosum
pT3	Tumor invades urethra
pT4	Tumor invades other adjacent structures
cN: Clinical definition of lymph node stage	
cNX	Regional lymph nodes cannot be assessed
cN0	No palpable or visibly enlarged inguinal lymph nodes
cN1	Palpable mobile unilateral inguinal lymph node
cN2	Palpable mobile multiple or bilateral inguinal lymph nodes
cN3	Palpable fixed inguinal nodal mass or pelvic lymphadenopathy unilateral or bilateral
pN: Pathologic lymph node stage	
pNX	Regional lymph nodes cannot be assessed
pN0	No regional lymph node metastasis
pN1	Metastasis in a single inguinal lymph node
pN2	Metastases in multiple or bilateral inguinal lymph nodes
pN3	Extranodal extension of lymph node metastasis or pelvic lymph node(s) unilateral or bilateral
M: Distant metastasis	
M0	No distant metastasis
M1	Distant metastasis

Stage groupings			
Stage	T	N	M
0	Tis	N0	M0
	Ta	N0	M0
I	T1a	N0	M0
II	T1b	N0	M0
	T2	N0	M0
	T3	N0	M0
IIIa	T1–3	N1	M0
IIIb	T1–3	N2	M0
IV	T4	Any N	M0
	Any T	N3	M0
	Any T	Any N	M1

Adapted from reference [50]

Used with the permission of the American Joint Committee on Cancer (AJCC), Chicago, Illinois. The original source for this material is the AJCC Cancer Staging Manual, Seventh Edition (2010), published by Springer Science and Business Media LLC, http://www.springer.com. Edge SB, Byrd DR, Compton CC, et al., editors. Penis. 7th ed. New York, NY: Springer; 2010

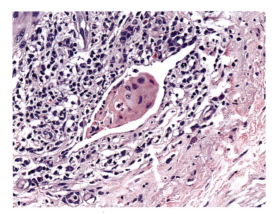

Fig. 3.24 Lymphovascular invasion by squamous cell carcinoma. H&E, 200×

Perineural Invasion

Perineural invasion has been reported to be present in between 33 and 50% of penile SCC specimens. Tumors with perineural invasion have been reported to be significantly associated with a worse prognosis [28, 48]. It should be noted that the diagnosis of perineural invasion should only be rendered when the tumor cells are surrounding the nerve and present within the perineural space, and should not be used for nerves that are only entrapped within the tumor. The penis has numerous nerves and the latter fact should be kept in mind when assessing for perineural invasion.

Role of Human Papilloma Virus in Penile Squamous Cell Carcinoma

The role of HPV, particularly subtypes 16 and 18, has been studied in squamous carcinomas of the penis, showing integration of the viral genome into tumor DNA [54, 55]. Wiener et al. were the first to describe the association between HPV and carcinomas of the male urethra, using a polymerase chain reaction (PCR)-based assay to detect the prevalence of HPV 16, 18, as well as nine additional low-risk HPV serotypes. They found a 29% incidence of HPV 16 in their subset of patients, with concordance between recurrent and metastatic disease in this patient population [56]. Since then, there have been several studies

that have attempted to reduplicate these efforts and currently it is believed that anywhere from 10 to 80% of penile SCCs are associated with HPV 16 or 18 [10, 56–58]. HPV 16 is the most common etiologic agent and accounts for approximately 60% of all HPV-positive histologic subtypes. HPV 16 has a particularly strong association with warty SCC as well as basaloid SCC. HPV18, despite being the second most prevalent HPV virus, has a much lower rate of prevalence and accounts for approximately 13% of all HPV-positive SCC [59]. The incidence of HPV detection varies depending on the SCC subtype, as has been discussed earlier in this chapter under the different subtypes. A PCR-based assay on formalin-fixed paraffin-embedded tissue is the most common methodology to assess HPV in the tumor tissue. Although the potential for false negative results or a failed assay due to DNA degradation exists, current literature suggests that this may be the most cost-effective approach. When fresh tissue is available, this may be used for PCR assays, although it is believed that there is no significant difference in detection rates amongst fresh frozen or paraffin-embedded tissue [59]. Current Center for Disease Control (CDC) data indicates that there are approximately 1,000 new cases of penile cancer diagnosed each year, of which approximately 36% are attributable to HPV [60]. The data suggest a potential future role for HPV vaccines in males and it is predicted that doing so is likely to reduce both the rate of infection as well as the incidence of HPV-related cancers in this patient population, especially in parts of the world with a high incidence of HPV infection [61].

Other Tumors of the Penis

While SCCs comprise most of the penile tumors seen in routine clinical practice, other tumor types that may involve the penis need to be kept in mind. Most tumors that involve the skin, subcutaneous tissue, and smooth muscle in other parts of the body have been reported to affect the penis, albeit in much smaller numbers considering that the penis is generally not sun-exposed.

Penile sarcomas are the second most common malignancy affecting the penis, yet they only comprise less than 5% of all penile malignancies. The incidence of penile sarcomas peaks in the fifth and sixth decades of life, except for embryonal rhabdomyosarcomas, which most commonly affect children [62, 63]. Most sarcomas involve the penile shaft, except for Kaposi's sarcoma, which most commonly occurs on the glans penis. Morphologic features of these sarcomas are similar to their counterparts arising in the soft tissue of other anatomical sites. Of all the sarcomas, vascular tumors are the most common, including Kaposi's sarcoma, epithelioid hemangioendothelioma, and angiosarcoma [64–66]. Leiomyosarcomas are the next most common sarcoma type, and may be either superficial or deep. Superficial leiomyosarcomas tend to form subcutaneous or submucosal nodules, originating from the corpus spongiosum of the glans penis or the dartos muscle or dermal smooth muscle of the penile shaft. The deep type is less common, originating from the smooth muscle of the corpora cavernosa, but is more aggressive with a tendency to invade the urethra and metastasize early [67].

Basal cell carcinoma involving the penile skin is uncommon, considering that the penile skin is generally not sun-exposed [68, 69]. Almost all reported cases have been in Caucasians, ranging in age at presentation from 37 to 79 years. These tumors most often involve the skin of the penile shaft, and less commonly the glans penis or the prepuce. These tumors typically present as a small, irregular, ulcerated mass. Morphologic features of these tumors are identical to basal cell carcinoma affecting the skin elsewhere. SCC with basaloid features is the main differential diagnostic consideration, as it is more common than basal cell carcinoma and is an aggressive tumor. As in other parts of the body, the clinical course of basal cell carcinoma is generally indolent, and these neoplasms may be treated by local excision alone without the need for a subsequent lymph node dissection.

Malignant melanoma of the penis is rare, with fewer than 200 reported cases [70, 71]. Melanoma tends to affect men in the fifth and sixth decades of life. Most tumors are located on the glans penis, with rare tumors arising on the foreskin and skin of the penile shaft. It should be noted that in some series, malignant melanomas affecting the penis and the penile urethra have been reported concomitantly. As with melanomas of the skin or mucosa, these tumors present as a pigmented plaque, macule, papule, or nodule that may enlarge within a few months. Some patients may have surface ulceration. Nodular, superficial spreading and acral lentiginous are the different morphologic types of malignant melanoma that have been reported. Malignant melanomas are typically treated by local excision, along with an inguinal lymph node dissection. Some centers use sentinel lymph node biopsy to decide on the necessity and extent of the inguinal lymph node dissection. Similar to melanomas elsewhere, prognosis is dependent on the depth of invasion and pathologic stage. Tumors invading at a depth <0.75 mm have a more favorable prognosis, while those invading >1.5 mm have a higher rate of metastases. Lentiginous melanosis, which is characterized by multiple flat pigmented macules on the glans penis, is a benign condition that should be included in the differential diagnosis of pigmented lesions on the glans penis [72].

Extra-mammary Paget's disease rarely affects the penis of older individuals. It presents as a red-tan plaque-like area on the skin, and may involve the penis and scrotum. Morphologic features are similar to those of other extra-mammary Paget's disease at other sites. The differential diagnosis includes SCC in situ and malignant melanoma [73]. Surgical excision of a wide area of skin with evaluation of surgical margins by frozen section analysis is often required to optimize local cancer control.

Metastases to the penis are rare, and do not usually pose a clinical diagnostic dilemma. Primary tumors reported to have metastasized to the penis include prostatic adenocarcinoma, colonic adenocarcinoma, urothelial carcinoma from the urinary bladder, and renal cell carcinoma [74, 75]. Metastatic tumors tend to invade and fill the vascular sinusoids of the corpora cavernosa and corpus spongiosum.

Conclusion

SCC is the most common tumor affecting the penis. Proper pathologic evaluation of penile tumors requires a working knowledge of the anatomy and histology of the penis, as the foreskin, glans penis, and penile shaft have different layers of tissue. Different terms have been used for premalignant squamous lesions of the penis, with PeIN being the latest proposed term. PeIN is divided into differentiated PeIN, which corresponds to mild and moderate squamous dysplasia, and undifferentiated PeIN, which corresponds to carcinoma in situ. The clinical manifestations of squamous carcinoma in situ include erythroplasia of Queyrat, Bowen's disease, and Bowenoid papulosis. SCCs of the penis most often originate on the glans penis, followed by the foreskin and penile shaft. These carcinomas most often show three patterns of growth (verruciform, superficial spreading, vertical), which are of prognostic importance. In addition to the usual type of SCC, which is morphologically similar to that seen in most squamous lined mucosas, there are other subtypes including papillary carcinoma NOS, warty carcinoma, verrucous carcinoma, basaloid carcinoma, mixed carcinomas, and carcinoma with sarcomatoid dedifferentiation, which have distinct morphologic features and prognostic significance. Other rare types of squamous carcinoma include mixed carcinoma, warty–basaloid carcinoma, adenosquamous carcinoma, pseudohyperplastic carcinoma, pseudoglandular carcinoma, and carcinoma cuniculatum. Predictive pathology features that need to be reported in penile SCC include histologic subtype, tumor grade, extent of invasion, lymphovascular invasion, perineural invasion, and TNM pathologic stage. HPV, particularly subtypes 16 and 18, have been implicated in the pathogenesis of penile SCC, especially in some subtypes such as warty and basaloid. Finally, tumors other than SCC may affect the penis, including sarcomas, malignant melanoma, basal cell carcinoma, and extramammary Paget's disease.

References

1. Cubilla AL, Piris A, Pfannl R, Rodriguez I, Aguero F, Young RH. Anatomic levels: important landmarks in penectomy specimens: a detailed anatomic and histologic study based on examination of 44 cases. Am J Surg Pathol. 2001;25(8):1091–4.
2. Velazquez EF, Barreto JE, Cold CJ, Cubilla AL. Penis and distal urethra. In: Mills SE, editor. Histology for Pathologists. Philadelphia, PA: Lippincott Williams & Wilkins; 2006. p. 965–80.
3. Grossman HB. Premalignant and early carcinomas of the penis and scrotum. Urol Clin North Am. 1992;19(2):221–6.
4. Horenblas S, von Krogh G, Cubilla AL, Dillner J, Meijer CJ, Hedlund PO. Squamous cell carcinoma of the penis: premalignant lesions. Scand J Urol Nephrol Suppl. 2000;205:187–8.
5. Cubilla AL, Meijer CJ, Young RH. Morphological features of epithelial abnormalities and precancerous lesions of the penis. Scand J Urol Nephrol Suppl. 2000;205:215–9.
6. Cubilla AL, Velazquez EF, Young RH. Epithelial lesions associated with invasive penile squamous cell carcinoma: a pathologic study of 288 cases. Int J Surg Pathol. 2004;12(4):351–64.
7. Velazquez EF, Chaux A, Cubilla AL. Histologic classification of penile intraepithelial neoplasia. Semin Diagn Pathol. 2012;29(2):96–102.
8. Chaux A, Pfannl R, Lloveras B, Alejo M, Clavero O, Lezcano C, et al. Distinctive association of p16INK4a overexpression with penile intraepithelial neoplasia depicting warty and/or basaloid features: a study of 141 cases evaluating a new nomenclature. Am J Surg Pathol. 2010;34(3):385–92.
9. Aynaud O, Ionesco M, Barrasso R. Penile intraepithelial neoplasia. Specific clinical features correlate with histologic and virologic findings. Cancer. 1994;74(6):1762–7.
10. Gregoire L, Cubilla AL, Reuter VE, Haas GP, Lancaster WD. Preferential association of human papillomavirus with high-grade histologic variants of penile-invasive squamous cell carcinoma. J Natl Cancer Inst. 1995;87(22):1705–9.
11. Graham JH, Helwig EB. Erythroplasia of Queyrat. A clinicopathologic and histochemical study. Cancer. 1973;32(6):1396–414.
12. Young RH, Srigley JR, Amin MB, Cubilla AL, Ulbright TM. The penis. In: Rosai J, Sobin LH, editors. Tumors and tumor-like lesions of the prostate, seminal vesicles, male urethra and penis Atlas of Tumor Pathology, series 3. Washington, D.C.: Armed Forces Institute of Pathology; 2000. p. 403–88.
13. Kaye V, Zhang G, Dehner LP, Fraley EE. Carcinoma in situ of penis. Is distinction between erythroplasia of Queyrat and Bowen's disease relevant? Urology. 1990;36(6):479–82.

14. Callen JP, Headington J. Bowen's and non-Bowen's squamous intraepidermal neoplasia of the skin. Relationship to internal malignancy. Arch Dermatol. 1980;116(4):422–6.
15. Taylor Jr DR, South DA. Bowenoid papulosis: a review. Cutis. 1981;27(1):92–8.
16. Patterson JW, Kao GF, Graham JH, Helwig EB. Bowenoid papulosis. A clinicopathologic study with ultrastructural observations. Cancer. 1986;57(4): 823–36.
17. Ikenberg H, Gissmann L, Gross G, Grussendorf-Conen EI, zur Hausen H. Human papillomavirus type-16-related DNA in genital Bowen's disease and in Bowenoid papulosis. Int J Cancer. 1983;32(5): 563–5.
18. Velazquez EF, Cubilla AL. Lichen sclerosus in 68 patients with squamous cell carcinoma of the penis: frequent atypias and correlation with special carcinoma variants suggests a precancerous role. Am J Surg Pathol. 2003;27(11):1448–53.
19. Fraley EE, Zhang G, Sazama R, Lange PH. Cancer of the penis. Prognosis and treatment plans. Cancer. 1985;55(7):1618–24.
20. Narayana AS, Olney LE, Loening SA, Weimar GW, Culp DA. Carcinoma of the penis: analysis of 219 cases. Cancer. 1982;49(10):2185–91.
21. Jones WG, Fossa SD, Hamers H, Van den Bogaert W. Penis cancer: a review by the Joint Radiotherapy Committee of the European Organisation for Research and Treatment of Cancer (EORTC) Genitourinary and Radiotherapy Groups. J Surg Oncol. 1989;40(4): 227–31.
22. Burgers JK, Badalament RA, Drago JR. Penile cancer. Clinical presentation, diagnosis, and staging. Urol Clin North Am. 1992;19(2):247–56.
23. Cubilla AL, Barreto J, Caballero C, Ayala G, Riveros M. Pathologic features of epidermoid carcinoma of the penis. A prospective study of 66 cases. Am J Surg Pathol. 1993;17(8):753–63.
24. Villavicencio H, Rubio-Briones J, Regalado R, Chechile G, Algaba F, Palou J. Grade, local stage and growth pattern as prognostic factors in carcinoma of the penis. Eur Urol. 1997;32(4):442–7.
25. Cubilla AL, Reuter V, Velazquez E, Piris A, Saito S, Young RH. Histologic classification of penile carcinoma and its relation to outcome in 61 patients with primary resection. Int J Surg Pathol. 2001;9(2): 111–20.
26. Cubilla AL, Velazques EF, Reuter VE, Oliva E, Mihm Jr MC, Young RH. Warty (condylomatous) squamous cell carcinoma of the penis: a report of 11 cases and proposed classification of 'verruciform' penile tumors. Am J Surg Pathol. 2000;24(4):505–12.
27. Velazquez EF, Soskin A, Bock A, Codas R, Barreto JE, Cubilla AL. Positive resection margins in partial penectomies: sites of involvement and proposal of local routes of spread of penile squamous cell carcinoma. Am J Surg Pathol. 2004;28(3):384–9.
28. Guimaraes GC, Cunha IW, Soares FA, Lopes A, Torres J, Chaux A, et al. Penile squamous cell carcinoma clinicopathological features, nodal metastasis and outcome in 333 cases. J Urol. 2009;182(2):528–34. Discussion 34.
29. Chaux A, Soares F, Rodriguez I, Barreto J, Lezcano C, Torres J, et al. Papillary squamous cell carcinoma, not otherwise specified (NOS) of the penis: clinico-pathologic features, differential diagnosis, and outcome of 35 cases. Am J Surg Pathol. 2010;34(2): 223–30.
30. Chaux A, Lezcano C, Cubilla AL, Tamboli P, Ro J, Ayala A. Comparison of subtypes of penile squamous cell carcinoma from high and low incidence geographical regions. Int J Surg Pathol. 2010;18(4): 268–77.
31. Bezerra AL, Lopes A, Landman G, Alencar GN, Torloni H, Villa LL. Clinicopathologic features and human papillomavirus dna prevalence of warty and squamous cell carcinoma of the penis. Am J Surg Pathol. 2001;25(5):673–8.
32. Johnson DE, Lo RK, Srigley J, Ayala AG. Verrucous carcinoma of the penis. J Urol. 1985;133(2):216–8.
33. Masih AS, Stoler MH, Farrow GM, Wooldridge TN, Johansson SL. Penile verrucous carcinoma: a clinicopathologic, human papillomavirus typing and flow cytometric analysis. Mod Pathol. 1992;5(1):48–55.
34. Kraus FT, Perez-Mesa C. Verrucous carcinoma: clinical and pathologic study of 105 cases involving oral cavity, larynx and genitalia. Cancer. 1966;19:26–38.
35. Robertson DI, Maung R, Duggan MA. Verrucous carcinoma of the genital tract: is it a distinct entity? Can J Surg. 1993;36(2):147–51.
36. Dai B, Ye DW, Kong YY, Yao XD, Zhang HL, Shen YJ. Predicting regional lymph node metastasis in Chinese patients with penile squamous cell carcinoma: the role of histopathological classification, tumor stage and depth of invasion. J Urol. 2006;176(4 (Pt 1)):1431–5. Discussion 5.
37. Cubilla AL, Reuter VE, Gregoire L, Ayala G, Ocampos S, Lancaster WD, et al. Basaloid squamous cell carcinoma: a distinctive human papilloma virus-related penile neoplasm: a report of 20 cases. Am J Surg Pathol. 1998;22(6):755–61.
38. Chaux A, Reuter V, Lezcano C, Velazquez EF, Torres J, Cubilla AL. Comparison of morphologic features and outcome of resected recurrent and nonrecurrent squamous cell carcinoma of the penis: a study of 81 cases. Am J Surg Pathol. 2009;33(9):1299–306.
39. Velazquez EF, Melamed J, Barreto JE, Aguero F, Cubilla AL. Sarcomatoid carcinoma of the penis: a clinicopathologic study of 15 cases. Am J Surg Pathol. 2005;29(9):1152–8.
40. Lont AP, Gallee MP, Snijders P, Horenblas S. Sarcomatoid squamous cell carcinoma of the penis: a clinical and pathological study of 5 cases. J Urol. 2004;172(3):932–5.
41. Kato N, Onozuka T, Yasukawa K, Kimura K, Sasaki K. Penile hybrid verrucous-squamous carcinoma associated with a superficial inguinal lymph node metastasis. Am J Dermatopathol. 2000;22(4): 339–43.

42. Chaux A, Tamboli P, Ayala A, Soares F, Rodriguez I, Barreto J, et al. Warty-basaloid carcinoma: clinico-pathological features of a distinctive penile neoplasm. Report of 45 cases. Mod Pathol. 2010;23(6): 896–904.

43. Cubilla AL, Ayala MT, Barreto JE, Bellasai JG, Noel JC. Surface adenosquamous carcinoma of the penis. A report of three cases. Am J Surg Pathol. 1996;20(2): 156–60.

44. Cubilla AL, Velazquez EF, Young RH. Pseudohyperplastic squamous cell carcinoma of the penis associated with lichen sclerosus. An extremely well-differentiated, nonverruciform neoplasm that preferentially affects the foreskin and is frequently misdiagnosed: a report of 10 cases of a distinctive clinicopathologic entity. Am J Surg Pathol. 2004;28(7): 895–900.

45. Cunha IW, Guimaraes GC, Soares F, Velazquez E, Torres JJ, Chaux A, et al. Pseudoglandular (adenoid, acantholytic) penile squamous cell carcinoma: a clini-copathologic and outcome study of 7 patients. Am J Surg Pathol. 2009;33(4):551–5.

46. Barreto JE, Velazquez EF, Ayala E, Torres J, Cubilla AL. Carcinoma cuniculatum: a distinctive variant of penile squamous cell carcinoma: report of 7 cases. Am J Surg Pathol. 2007;31(1):71–5.

47. Velazquez EF, Ayala G, Liu H, Chaux A, Zanotti M, Torres J, et al. Histologic grade and perineural inva-sion are more important than tumor thickness as pre-dictor of nodal metastasis in penile squamous cell carcinoma invading 5 to 10 mm. Am J Surg Pathol. 2008;32(7):974–9.

48. Chaux A, Torres J, Pfannl R, Barreto J, Rodriguez I, Velazquez EF, et al. Histologic grade in penile squamous cell carcinoma: visual estimation versus digital measurement of proportions of grades, adverse prognosis with any proportion of grade 3 and correla-tion of a Gleason-like system with nodal metastasis. Am J Surg Pathol. 2009;33(7):1042–9.

49. Slaton JW, Morgenstern N, Levy DA, Santos Jr MW, Tamboli P, Ro JY, et al. Tumor stage, vascular inva-sion and the percentage of poorly differentiated can-cer: independent prognosticators for inguinal lymph node metastasis in penile squamous cancer. J Urol. 2001;165(4):1138–42.

50. Edge SB, Byrd DR, Compton CC, et al. (editors). Penis. 7th ed. New York, NY: Springer; 2010

51. Leijte JA, Gallee M, Antonini N, Horenblas S. Evaluation of current TNM classification of penile carcinoma. J Urol. 2008;180(3):933–8. Discussion 8.

52. Lopes A, Bezerra AL, Pinto CA, Serrano SV, de Mell OC, Villa LL. p53 as a new prognostic factor for lymph node metastasis in penile carcinoma: analysis of 82 patients treated with amputation and bilateral lymphadenectomy. J Urol. 2002;168(1):81–6.

53. Ficarra V, Martignoni G, Maffei N, Cerruto MA, Novara G, Cavalleri S, et al. Predictive pathological factors of lymph nodes involvement in the squamous

cell carcinoma of the penis. Int Urol Nephrol. 2002;34(2):245–50.

54. Kalantari M, Villa LL, Calleja-Macias IE, Bernard HU. Human papillomavirus-16 and -18 in penile car-cinomas: DNA methylation, chromosomal recombi-nation and genomic variation. Int J Cancer. 2008;123(8):1832–40.

55. Rubin MA, Kleter B, Zhou M, Ayala G, Cubilla AL, Quint WG, et al. Detection and typing of human pap-illomavirus DNA in penile carcinoma: evidence for multiple independent pathways of penile carcinogen-esis. Am J Pathol. 2001;159(4):1211–8.

56. Wiener JS, Effert PJ, Humphrey PA, Yu L, Liu ET, Walther PJ. Prevalence of human papillomavirus types 16 and 18 in squamous-cell carcinoma of the penis: a retrospective analysis of primary and meta-static lesions by differential polymerase chain reac-tion. Int J Cancer. 1992;50(5):694–701.

57. Chan KW, Lam KY, Chan AC, Lau P, Srivastava G. Prevalence of human papillomavirus types 16 and 18 in penile carcinoma: a study of 41 cases using PCR. J Clin Pathol. 1994;47(9):823–6.

58. Krustrup D, Jensen HL, van den Brule AJ, Frisch M. Histological characteristics of human papilloma-virus-positive and -negative invasive and in situ squamous cell tumours of the penis. Int J Exp Pathol. 2009;90(2):182–9.

59. Miralles-Guri C, Bruni L, Cubilla AL, Castellsague X, Bosch FX, de Sanjose S. Human papillomavirus prevalence and type distribution in penile carcinoma. J Clin Pathol. 2009;62(10):870–8.

60. Centers for Disease Control and Prevention (CDC). Human papillomavirus-associated cancers—United States, 2004–2008. MMWR Morb Mortal Wkly Rep. 2012;61:258–61.

61. Anderson LA. Prophylactic human papillomavirus vaccines: past, present and future. Pathology. 2012;44(1):1–6.

62. Dehner LP, Smith BH. Soft tissue tumors of the penis. A clinicopathologic study of 46 cases. Cancer. 1970;25(6):1431–47.

63. Dalkin B, Zaontz MR. Rhabdomyosarcoma of the penis in children. J Urol. 1989;141(4):908–9.

64. Weiss SW, Enzinger FM. Epithelioid hemangioen-dothelioma: a vascular tumor often mistaken for a carcinoma. Cancer. 1982;50(5):970–81.

65. Rasbridge SA, Parry JR. Angiosarcoma of the penis. Br J Urol. 1989;63(4):440–1.

66. Skoog SJ, Belman AB. Aphallia: its classification and management. J Urol. 1989;141(3):589–92.

67. Isa SS, Almaraz R, Magovern J. Leiomyosarcoma of the penis. Case report and review of the literature. Cancer. 1984;54(5):939–42.

68. McGregor DH, Tanimura A, Weigel JW. Basal cell carcinoma of penis. Urology. 1982;20(3):320–3.

69. Goldminz D, Scott G, Klaus S. Penile basal cell carci-noma. Report of a case and review of the literature. J Am Acad Dermatol. 1989;20(6):1094–7.

70. Oldbring J, Mikulowski P. Malignant melanoma of the penis and male urethra. Report of nine cases and review of the literature. Cancer. 1987;59(3):581–7.

71. Sanchez-Ortiz R, Huang SF, Tamboli P, Prieto VG, Hester G, Pettaway CA. Melanoma of the penis, scrotum and male urethra: a 40-year single institution experience. J Urol. 2005;173(6):1958–65.

72. Barnhill RL, Albert LS, Shama SK, Goldenhersh MA, Rhodes AR, Sober AJ. Genital lentiginosis: A clinical and histopathologic study. J Am Acad Dermatol. 1990;22:453–60.

73. Mitsudo S, Nakanishi I, Koss LG. Paget's disease of the penis and adjacent skin: its association with fatal sweat gland carcinoma. Arch Pathol Lab Med. 1981;105(10):518–20.

74. Philip AT, Amin MB, Cubilla AL, et al. Secondary tumors of the penis: A study of 16 cases. Mod Pathol. 1999;12:104A.

75. Chaux A, Amin M, Cubilla AL, Young RH. Metastatic tumors to the penis: a report of 17 cases and review of the literature. Int J Surg Pathol. 2011;19(5): 597–606.

Evolving Imaging Modalities in the Diagnosis and Staging of Penile Cancer

Adam S. Feldman and W. Scott McDougal

Introduction

Accurate staging of penile cancer is of paramount importance in the evaluation of a patient with penile cancer and the development of its optimal treatment plan. Squamous cell carcinoma (SCC) of the penis has a relatively predictable pattern of metastatic spread via the lymphatic system. It is this reliable pattern of spread which makes this disease one of the rare malignancies in which a thorough and effective resection of regional lymphatic involvement can result in potential cure. Metastatic spread of SCC from the penis first involves the superficial and deep inguinal lymph nodes, followed by the pelvic lymph nodes. The presence of metastatic disease in the regional lymph nodes and the extent of lymph node involvement are vital determinants of patient survival. Local staging of penile cancer and an understanding of the invasiveness and extent of the primary tumor are also essential for adequate surgical planning. Adequate preoperative assessment of local clinical staging allows for effective decision making for penile sparing surgery

(partial penectomy, wide local excision) versus the necessity for a more radical local resection. Moreover, it allows a frank discussion with the patient as to what can be expected postoperatively. A detailed discussion of the postsurgical appearance of the external genitalia is critical for the patient's psychological well-being. Therefore, the ability to accurately stage the local and regional extent of disease is paramount for the effective management of penile cancer.

Staging of the Primary Tumor

Although thoroughly discussed in a prior chapter of this book (see Chap. 2), the current staging of penile cancer follows the tumor, nodes, metastasis (TNM) staging system. For penile cancer, this was originally developed in 1978 and was most recently revised in 2009 by the American joint committee on cancer (AJCC) [1]. For the local tumor staging, this system describes the primary tumor and its relationship or possible invasion of local anatomical structures within and/or adjacent to the penis. Classification of the primary tumor in the TNM system ranges as follows: Tis: carcinoma in situ; Ta: noninvasive verrucous carcinoma; T1a: tumor which invades in the subepithelial connective tissue without lymphovascular invasion (LVI) and is not poorly differentiated (i.e., Grade 3–4); T1b: tumor which invades the subepithelial connective tissue with LVI or is poorly differentiated; T2: tumor which invades

A.S. Feldman, M.D., M.P.H. (✉)
W.S. McDougal, M.D.
Department of Urology, Massachusetts General Hospital, 55 Fruit St., Yawkey 7E, Boston, MA 02114, USA
e-mail: afeldman@partners.org

the corpus spongiosum or cavernosum; T3: tumor which invades the urethra; and T4: tumor invading other adjacent structures.

Although the true pathologic stage of the primary tumor is ultimately determined following surgical resection, an effective clinical determination of local tumor staging preoperatively is imperative. An estimation of the local extent of the primary tumor is necessary to determine the most suitable form of surgical resection. For larger tumors, a distinction must be made between the ability to perform a partial penectomy, subtotal penectomy, or radical penectomy. For smaller, more isolated tumors the selection of patients for penile sparing surgery must be considered. An accurate assessment of the depth of tumor invasion prior to resection can help better select appropriate patients for a successful outcome with such a penile sparing approach. We have found that invasive tumors ($\geq$T2) are not properly treated with penile sparing surgery and these patients should not be candidates for this approach [2].

In addition to the benefit for preoperative planning, accurate early clinical staging can potentially improve prognosis and minimize the risk of metastatic progression. It has been well demonstrated in the literature that invasion ($\geq$T2), poorly differentiated cells (Grade 3 or 4), or LVI are all predictors of regional lymph node involvement and therefore survival [3–10]. Thus, effective clinical staging at the time of tumor detection can be very helpful in providing patients with an outlook of their treatment options with their imparted prognosis.

Physical Examination

The initial staging of a patient with penile cancer begins with a proper physical examination. As per the 2009 European Association of Urology (EAU) Penile Cancer Guidelines, a physical examination should include the diameter of the penile lesion(s) or suspicious area(s), the location and number of lesion(s), the morphology of the lesion(s), the relationship of the lesion(s) to other structures, the color and boundaries of the lesion(s), and the penile length and expected

residual length if a partial penectomy is to be performed [11]. Clinical examination can be very helpful in assessing the primary tumor stage and can be helpful in estimating the extent of tumor invasion. When a lesion is on the penile shaft, one can assess for fixation versus mobility of the skin from the underlying tissue layers, corpora cavernosa, and/or urethra. Physical examination of lesions on the glans penis can potentially be more difficult to accurately assess. Lont et al. [12] previously demonstrated the high accuracy of the physical examination for detecting invasion of the corpora cavernosa, with a sensitivity of 86%, specificity of 100%, and positive predictive value of 100%. Petralia et al. [13, 14] demonstrated a slightly lower accuracy of the physical examination with 3 of 12 patients understaged and 2 of 12 patients overstaged.

Imaging for Staging of Primary Tumor

Although it is not our routine practice to obtain imaging for primary tumor staging (as discussed earlier), there are clinical circumstances in which this additional information can be beneficial. For historical purposes, the use of cavernosography is worth mentioning. This technique is performed by the direct injection of radiographic contrast media into the corpora cavernosa with the intent of demonstrating potential filling defects resulting from malignant lesions. This method has been used in the evaluation of local invasion of the corpora cavernosa by penile tumors [14] as well as in the metastatic spread to the corpora cavernosa from other neoplasms [15, 16]. The use of cavernosography, however, has been replaced by the use of more modern imaging modalities which are noninvasive and can also evaluate surrounding anatomical structures.

Ultrasound
Ultrasound is a readily available, noninvasive imaging technique for the evaluation of the primary penile tumor. Ultrasound evaluation of the penis can often delineate the specific tissue planes within the shaft of the penis including the urethra, corpus spongiosum, corpus cavernosum,

and tunica albuginea [17]. Horenblas et al. [18] assessed the ability of ultrasound to predict local tumor staging and correlated preoperative imaging with histopathology. Tumors were visualized as hypoechoic lesions on ultrasound and along the shaft of the penis and could be distinguished from the urethra, tunica albuginea, and corpora cavernosa. Although the presence of corpora cavernosum invasion could be accurately demonstrated in larger lesions on the shaft of the penis, invasion by lesions isolated to the glans was less effectively identified by ultrasound. This method could not reliably differentiate invasion of the subepithelial tissue from invasion of the corpus spongiosum.

Ultrasound evaluation of the primary tumor as a possible adjunct to physical examination was suggested in the 2004 EAU Guidelines on Penile Cancer as the preferred method of imaging for suspected invasion of the corpus cavernosum [19]. Interestingly however, the newly revised 2009 EAU Guidelines on Penile Cancer do not mention utilizing penile ultrasonography for this purpose [11]. These updated guidelines instead recommend the possible use of magnetic resonance imaging (MRI) to help identify the depth of invasion of the primary penile tumor.

Magnetic Resonance Imaging

MRI is an effective imaging modality for visualization of the anatomical structures of the penis and surrounding structures. It provides excellent soft tissue resolution and contrast within the layers of the penis and demonstrates a relatively clear delineation of the fascial planes and corporal bodies of the penis. The normal penile anatomy is composed of three cylindrical bodies which travel lengthwise along the shaft of the penis. The two erectile bodies or corpora cavernosa lie adjacent to one another dorsally, and then deviate laterally at the crus of the penis where they attach to the ischiopubic rami. The corpus spongiosum, which contains the penile and bulbar urethra, lies ventral to the corpora cavernosa and then extends distally and anteriorly to form the glans penis. These three cylindrical structures are covered independently by the tunica albuginea, and are then held together within Buck's

fascia. Superficial to Buck's fascia lies a layer of subcutaneous connective tissue, followed by dartos fascia exterior to this, and lastly covered by the overlying skin of the penis.

Both Buck's fascia and the tunica albuginea are visualized on both T1- and T2-weighted images as a single low-intensity layer of tissue surrounding the corporal bodies and therefore are indistinguishable from one another. They are, however, very distinguishable from the overlying subcutaneous connective tissue, and more importantly for staging purposes, distinct from both the corpora cavernosa and corpus spongiosum [20]. This ability of MRI to accurately distinguish these respective layers provides an effective imaging modality for local penile tumor clinical staging.

There are several techniques which can improve the quality of MRI imaging of the penis and its surrounding structures. To reduce motion artifact during image acquisition, the penis can be placed in the anatomic position and taped to the suprapubic region which helps to fix the penis in a constant position throughout the study [21]. A surface radiofrequency coil may also be placed over the penis to help improve the signal-to-noise ratio and provide finer anatomical imaging of the penis [22]. Penile tumors appear on MRI as a hypointense lesion(s) and are best evaluated on T2-weighted images which provide excellent resolution between the hypointense tumor(s) and fascial layers and the hyperintense corpora (Fig. 4.1). Gadolinium contrast tends to be less helpful in assessing for corporal invasion given that the corporal bodies normally enhance quite significantly and therefore can make tumor characterization less optimal [23].

Another technical method which has been studied to improve the ability of MRI for local staging of penile tumors is with intracavernosal injection of prostaglandin E1 (alprostadil) for the purposes of producing penile erection during the study [23]. The rationale behind this method is that in the flaccid penis there may be greater difficulty in assessing the corporal bodies, particularly if there is intracavernosal fibrosis resulting in a low T2 signal intensity and a reduction of the fine interface between the tunica albuginea and the corpora cavernosa. The induced penile

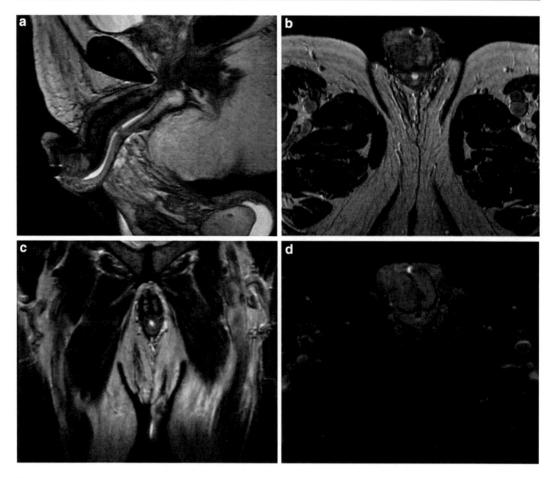

Fig. 4.1 MRI imaging of penile tumor for local staging purposes. (**a**) The mass in the distal shaft of the penis can be seen invading the corpora cavernosum and impinging the urethra in this T2-weighted sagittal image. (**b**) This T2-weighted axial image demonstrates the tumor invading the right corpora cavernosum and crossing the midline into the left corporal body. (**c**) This coronal image demonstrates the uninvolved bulbar urethra, proximal corpora cavernosa, and bony pelvis. (**d**) T1-weighted post-gadolinium images demonstrate tumor enhancement, but also enhancement of the corpora cavernosa

erection increases the size of the phallus, thereby improving imaging details and producing an increased blood flow within the corpora cavernosa, resulting in a greater signal intensity and contrast within the tunica.

This method of pharmacologically induced penile erection for MRI has been studied and compared with clinical staging by physical examination to predict local penile tumor stage determined pathologically. Petralia et al. [13] reported their experience with the use of intracavernosal prostaglandin E1 in 13 patients. This method of MRI image acquisition correctly staged 12 of 13 patients. In the one patient who was understaged by this method, MRI failed to identify *carcinoma*

in situ at the coronal sulcus. These results were compared with physical examination by which only 8 of the 13 patients were correctly staged. The five patients who were incorrectly staged by physical examination alone had tumors involving the glans and/or foreskin. Tumor location did not affect the ability of the MRI technique to correctly stage tumors, and therefore it may be that MRI has the greatest clinical benefit in assessing the preoperative clinical stage of primary penile tumors situated on the glans and/or foreskin.

Unfortunately the combination of pharmacologically induced penile erection with MRI has not been directly compared with the use of standard MRI alone and therefore it is not clear exactly how additionally valuable the use of intracavernosal agent has been. This certainly must be considered given the potential risk of intracavernosal injections (i.e., priapism, fibrosis, pain). Additionally, the true utility and advantage of preoperative imaging to predict local pathologic staging must be weighed against the inherent cost of such studies. Clearly preoperative imaging is not needed for every penile tumor prior to excision. However, accurate preoperative staging can be helpful in larger tumors which may extend more deeply into adjacent structures. This can help the surgeon determine resectability of a tumor and help counsel patients on their expected treatment outcomes and the extent of resection anticipated. Based on the imaging modalities currently available, when appropriate, MRI appears to be the imaging modality of choice for primary penile tumor clinical staging.

Staging of the Regional Lymph Nodes

The primary metastatic spread of penile carcinoma occurs via the regional lymphatic system, first spreading to the inguinal lymph node groups and then to the iliac and pelvic lymphatic chains. Due to the coalescence and frequent crossover patterns of the lymphatic channels at the base of the penis, lymphatic drainage from the penis to the inguinal nodal region occurs to both the superficial and deep inguinal nodes bilaterally irrespective of the location of the primary tumor. This lymphatic anatomy at the base of the penis which results in crossover lymphatic drainage may impair the surgeon's ability to determine the laterality of nodal metastases [24].

Despite this concern, penile cancer does generally spread in a dependable and sequential fashion to the inguinal region with subsequent drainage to the pelvic nodes. Multiple series have also demonstrated that the presence of lymph node metastases and the extent of nodal involvement are the most important predictors of patient survival [3, 25, 26]. Therefore, penile cancer is one of the uncommon malignancies in which a thorough resection of regional lymphatic involvement can result in cure. For this reason,

the ability to accurately and effectively assess the regional lymph node involvement is critical in the decision making and management of penile cancer.

Physical Examination

At the time of initial presentation of penile cancer, approximately half of all patients will have palpable inguinal lymphadenopathy on physical exam. Of all patients with palpable adenopathy at presentation, approximately 50% will be found to harbor metastatic disease. Due to infection or inflammatory change associated with the primary tumor, the other half of these men will have benign palpable adenopathy [27]. In an effort to reduce the number of falsely positive clinical exam findings of inguinal adenopathy, it is standard practice to place such patients on 2–6 weeks of antibiotic therapy following resection of the primary lesion and to reassess for resolution of the palpable nodes after a few weeks [19]. Persistently palpable inguinal adenopathy after 4–6 weeks of appropriate antibiotic therapy is most often consistent with metastatic disease. Similarly, the development of new adenopathy during follow-up is also a predictive sign of metastatic involvement of the inguinal lymph nodes.

In addition to the risk of false positives on physical examination, there is also a significant risk of a false-negative physical examination. Multiple series have demonstrated that the absence of palpable inguinal adenopathy is not sufficient for absolutely ruling out metastatic involvement; approximately 25% (range 11–62%) of patients without palpable inguinal adenopathy will harbor microscopic metastatic disease [4, 6, 26, 28, 29].

Pathologic Features of the Primary Tumor as a Predictor of Regional Lymph Node Involvement

Due to the high risk of false negatives in determining lymph node involvement by physical examination alone, an accurate ability to effectively predict regional nodal microscopic metastases has been an important goal over the past two decades. It has been demonstrated that the risk of regional lymph node involvement can be stratified by the histopathologic characteristics of the primary tumor. McDougal et al. [3] demonstrated that in patients with no palpable inguinal lymphadenopathy, invasion of the primary tumor into the corporal bodies suggested a significantly higher risk for metastatic involvement of the inguinal nodes. Horenblas et al. [4] also demonstrated that primary tumors which were of high grade or poorly differentiated resulted in a greater risk for nodal metastases.

In 1995, McDougal demonstrated that the combination of tumor invasion and microscopic cellular differentiation significantly improved the prediction of inguinal node metastases. This analysis demonstrated that of all patients whose tumors demonstrated corporal invasion or poorly differentiated cells, 83% were found to have regional lymph node involvement. Of those patients with poorly differentiated tumors or corporal invasion and who had nonpalpable nodes, 78% still had microscopic metastatic disease. These numbers can be compared with only a 4% risk of nodal metastases in those patients with moderately to well-differentiated tumor and no evidence of corporal invasion [5].

Corporal body invasion and poor cellular differentiation have been confirmed by several studies as predictive indicators for regional lymph node involvement [6–9]. In addition to these two determinants, the presence of LVI has also been identified in multiple studies as a predictor of lymph node metastases [6, 10, 30]. Based on these pathologic indicators, the 2009 revision of the AJCC penile cancer staging sub-stratified pT1 disease into pT1a: tumor which invades the subepithelial connective tissue without LVI and is not poorly differentiated (i.e., Grade 3 or 4) and pT1b: tumor which invades the subepithelial connective tissue with LVI or is poorly differentiated [1]. In addition, many groups view the presence of corporal invasion (pT2) or poorly differentiated cells (even in pT1 disease) as indicators for the necessity of preemptive inguinal lymphadenectomy in patients with clinically node negative disease.

Imaging for Staging of the Regional Lymph Nodes

Although current operative techniques have been refined to reduce the risk of complications from a radical inguinal lymph node dissection, there still remains a risk of perioperative and postoperative morbidity including wound infection, wound dehiscence/skin edge necrosis, deep venous thrombosis, neuropraxia/nerve injury, vascular injury/hematoma, lymphocele, and lower extremity lymphedema [31]. Given the risk of false positives and negatives with physical examination of the inguinal region, as well as the risk of overtreatment with lymphadenectomy among some patients with high-risk pathologic features as discussed earlier, effective imaging modalities of regional lymph nodes for more accurate staging of both macroscopic and microscopic disease are sought as they could significantly improve patient care and management strategies.

Ultrasound and Fine Needle Aspiration

Ultrasound with or without fine needle aspiration (FNA) has been utilized effectively as a diagnostic tool in other malignancies. Ultrasound evaluation of lymph nodes includes assessment of the node size, shape, and specific characteristics of echogenicity. Suspicious nodes demonstrate a rounded shape with a long and short axis diameter ratio of less than two, loss of hilar fat, and increased thickness or low echogenicity in the nodal cortex [32, 33]. Using color Doppler evaluation of nodal perfusion, metastatic nodes often demonstrate peripheral vascularity while reactive nodes demonstrate an increased pattern of hilar perfusion [34].

Ultrasound by itself has been demonstrated to be an inadequate evaluation of clinically negative inguinal lymph nodes, with a sensitivity of 74%, specificity of 77%, and positive predicted value of 37% [35]. The combination of FNA with ultrasound to biopsy suspicious-appearing nodes has also been demonstrated to have unsatisfactory results, with a sensitivity of 39% and a specificity of 100%. These data demonstrate the inadequacy of this method for the effective evaluation of inguinal lymph node involvement in the absence of palpable adenopathy.

In the case of clinically palpable inguinal adenopathy, the 2009 EAU Guidelines recommend FNA as an option for the evaluation of palpable nodes at presentation of disease [11]. Due to the knowledge that 50% of clinically palpable nodes at presentation will be due to inflammatory reaction/infection, our algorithm in this scenario has been to place patients on appropriate antibiotic therapy and reevaluate at 4 weeks. Those with persistent adenopathy after 4–6 weeks on antibiotics undergo an inguinal lymph node dissection.

Cross-sectional Imaging

Cross-sectional imaging using either computed tomography (CT) or MRI can detect bulky lymphadenopathy. These imaging techniques, however, depend only on the size and morphology of lymph nodes to assess their potential malignant phenotype. Even the experienced radiologist may be unable to effectively distinguish between malignant and benign nodal enlargement in many cases, resulting in the potential for significant false positives. Furthermore, given the reliance on the nodal size as the major measurable factor, conventional CT and MRI cannot detect microscopic metastatic disease in normal sized and appearing lymph nodes. Conventional MRI parameters have been demonstrated to have unsatisfactory results in the detection of lymph node metastases, with a sensitivity and specificity of 13 and 76%, respectively [36].

A recent study investigated the ability of conventional CT to identify patients with inguinal node involvement with high-risk features, defined as ≥3 nodes involved, extranodal extension, and/or pelvic lymph node involvement on histopathologic analysis [37]. This study evaluated various CT features, and demonstrated that the finding of central nodal necrosis and/or the presence of an irregular nodal border could predict high-risk lymph node involvement with a sensitivity of 95% and a specificity of 82%. The sensitivity of detecting pelvic nodal involvement, however, was only 20%. Even using these specific imaging parameters, CT did result in a high false-negative rate in predicting any pathologic nodal involvement (i.e., low and high risk). Nevertheless,

the authors discuss that the use of these features may help to identify patients with pathologic high-risk features of lymph node involvement and who may benefit from neoadjuvant systemic chemotherapy.

Lymphotrophic Nanoparticle-Enhanced MRI

Although conventional MRI provides excellent soft tissue resolution, it is still very much dependent on the evaluation of nodal size and shape in assessing for possible metastatic involvement. Lymphotrophic nanoparticle-enhanced MRI (LNMRI) is a novel method for evaluating lymph nodes for metastatic spread of penile cancer and other malignancies. This technique utilizes ultrasmall superparamagnetic iron oxide (USPIO) particles, which are composed of a biodegradable monocrystalline, inverse spinel iron oxide core, and a polymer coating composed of low-molecular-weight dextran. The entire nanoparticle ranges in size from 30 to 50 nm and the iron oxide core measures 4.3–6.0 nm [38].

These particles represent a new class of MRI contrast agents, which were initially developed for imaging of the liver. When it became evident that the USPIO particles were able to pass across capillary walls, systemically localize into lymph nodes, and allow for characterization of lymph nodes independent of size, investigations began into their ability to assess for metastatic lymph node involvement of multiple malignancies [39, 40]. These particles localize to lymph nodes by two mechanisms, the major pathway being by direct trans-capillary passage from the venules within the medullary sinuses of lymph nodes, and the secondary pathway being via the local lymphatic drainage system after extravasation within tissue capillary beds (Fig. 4.2).

In the lymph node, the nanoparticles are phagocytosed and accumulated within macrophages of the reticuloendothelial system (RES). In benign nodes, with an intact and homogeneous RES, the deposition of these nanoparticles results in a drop in the T2 signal intensity. Complete or partial infiltration of lymph nodes with malignant cells displaces the macrophages of the RES with lack of uptake of USPIO particles and therefore causes

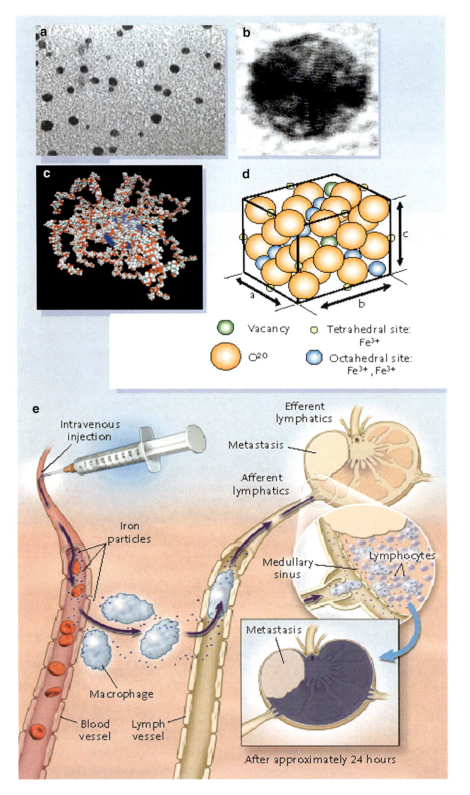

Fig. 4.2 (**a**, **b**) Electron micrograph of USPIO particles. The mean size of the nanoparticles is 2–3 nm on average (**c**, **d**). Molecular model of the 10 kDa dextrans and iron oxide crystal. The mean particle size of the 10 kDa dextrans is 28 nm. (**e**) Mechanism of action of lymphotrophic nanoparticle. From N Engl J Med, Harisinghani MG, Barentsz J, Hahn PF, Deserno WM, Tabatabaei S, van de Kaa CH, et al., Noninvasive detection of clinically occult lymph-node metastases in prostate cancer, 348(25), pp. 2491–9. Copyright © 2003 Massachusetts Medical Society. Reprinted with permission from Massachusetts Medical Society

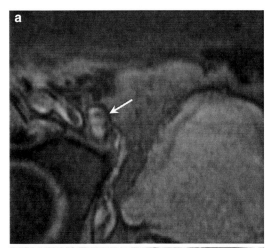

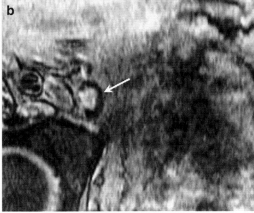

Fig. 4.3 Histopathologically demonstrated 11 mm metastatic right inguinal lymph node. (**a**) T2 image, pre-contrast, demonstrates bright (*arrow*) node. (**b**) 24 h post ferumoxtran-10, no decrease in signal is seen suggesting metastatic deposit which was demonstrated by pathology of that node. Reprinted from J Urol, 174(3), Tabatabaei S, Harisinghani M, McDougal WS, Regional lymph node staging using lymphotropic nanoparticle enhanced magnetic resonance imaging with ferumoxtran-10 in patients with penile cancer, pp. 923–927, Copyright (2005), with permission from Elsevier

these nodes to retain a bright or heterogeneous image on the post-contrast phase of the imaging study (Fig. 4.3) [41, 42]. Using this technique, false-positive results may result from nodal fibrosis, granulomatous change or other infectious causes, lymph node necrosis, or insufficiency in a particle dose [43–45]. False-negative interpretations may occur when microscopic foci of metastatic cells are below the detection limit and resolution of current MRI technology [46].

The utility of LNMRI was evaluated in seven patients with SCC of the penis as a preoperative assessment before planned bilateral radical inguinal lymphadenectomy [36]. Radiologic and pathologic correlation was assessed postoperatively. There were a total of 113 lymph nodes evaluated, with 100 benign and 13 malignant. The sensitivity and specificity of conventional MRI using size criteria for the detection of nodal metastatic disease were 13 and 76%, respectively. Of the 13 malignant nodes, only 3 met the size criteria by standard MRI evaluation, and 13% of the histologically benign nodes exceeded the standard MRI size criteria of a short axis diameter >10 mm. Using LNMRI in this same group resulted in a sensitivity of 100% and a specificity of 97% for the detection of metastases in individual lymph nodes, with a positive predictive value of 81.2% and a negative predictive value of 100%.

The original investigations of USPIO particles utilized Ferumoxtran-10 (Combidex [Advanced Magnetics, Cambridge, MA], Sinerem [Laboratorie Guerbet, Aulnay-sous-Bois, France]). Unfortunately in 2005, in spite of encouraging data in multiple malignancies, Ferumoxtran-10 did not receive FDA approval. Since that time the next generation of USPIO particles, Ferumoxytol (Feraheme [AMAG Pharmaceuticals, Lexington, MA]), has been developed with a carboxymethyl dextran coating, which allows for greater iron concentration, minimizes allergic side effects, and has an improved safety profile. This new agent is currently being investigated and it is hoped that it will have the same promising results as its predecessor.

Positron Emission Tomography–Computed Tomography

Positron emission tomography (PET) using fluorine-18-fluorodeoxyglucose (18F-FDG) allows for functional imaging of malignant cells based on tumor cellular metabolism. This imaging technique is based on the elevated glycolytic rate of malignant cells and demonstrates areas with enhanced cellular uptake of glucose and 18F-FDG [47]. In order to enhance the utility of the data acquired from PET imaging, PET–CT scanners have become readily available and fuse the

PET and CT data acquired from a single scanner into a single image containing both functional and anatomic information. The use of this combined technique has been demonstrated to be quite helpful in other malignancies, with an improved accuracy over either PET or CT alone [48–50].

Scher et al. [51] first evaluated PET–CT in the evaluation of penile cancer patients who were suspected of having recurrent disease. In 13 men, the sensitivity of detecting lymph node metastases was 80% and specificity was 100%. The authors also noted that in regard to the detection of metastases within inguinal/pelvic lymph nodes, the sensitivity was 89% for superficial inguinal lymph nodes and 100% for metastases in the deep inguinal and obturator nodes. Graafland et al. [52] assessed PT–CT in 21 patients with penile cancer with cytologically demonstrated inguinal lymph node metastases. In this group, all patients with cytologically and clinically positive inguinal adenopathy demonstrated increased FDG uptake in those regions. They further identified that PET–CT had a sensitivity of 91% and a specificity of 100% for detecting pelvic nodal involvement.

This same group also assessed 24 patients with clinically negative inguinal nodes (cN0) [53]. In this cohort of patients, the results were much less encouraging. Only one of five patients with pathologically positive inguinal lymph node involvement was correctly identified by PET–CT, resulting in a sensitivity of only 20%. All of the false-negative studies resulted in patients with metastatic deposits ≤10 mm. Souillac et al. [54] also assessed the utility of PET–CT and within their study had 22 cases of cN0 disease. In these clinically node negative patients, the sensitivity for detection of inguinal nodal involvement was 75% with a specificity of 87.5%. Although these results for cN0 disease are slightly more encouraging than the previous study, these data still do question the ability of PET–CT to dependably rule out microscopic metastatic deposits in the inguinal lymph nodes in this patient subset.

A recent systematic review and meta-analysis further investigated the utility of PET–CT [55]. This evaluation which compiled and analyzed the data from seven previously published studies noted that while in clinically node-positive disease the sensitivity and specificity were 96 and 100%, respectively, in clinically node-negative disease, the sensitivity was 56% and the specificity was 86%. These results support the concerns that 18F-FDG-PT–CT is inadequate for assessing patients with cN0 disease when making decisions about early inguinal lymphadenectomy.

Dynamic Lymphoscintigraphy and Sentinel Lymph Node Biopsy

Due to the concerns of the risk of the added morbidity from inguinal lymphadenectomy in clinically node-negative patients, several groups have attempted to reduce the number of radical groin dissections performed with techniques to identify those with nodal metastases by limiting the need and extent of surgical exploration. The concept of a sentinel node is one which identifies a specific node or subgroup of nodes to which the primary lymphatic drainage from the penis occurs. It has been suggested in the past that the sentinel node in the inguinal region for penile cancer resides adjacent to the superficial epigastric vein and would be predictive of the status of the inguinal nodes [56, 57]. These original descriptions, however, did not clearly depict false-negative measurements. In addition, the sentinel node's precise location likely varies from patient to patient, and the reproducibility of this original description has been proven unreliable by several groups [58–61].

Based on this concept, an effort has been made to improve the accuracy of this method taking into account the patient-to-patient variability in the precise location of the sentinel lymph node. Intraoperative lymph node mapping or a dynamic sentinel lymph node biopsy (DSNB) has been proposed based on positive experiences in both the breast cancer and melanoma scientific literature [62]. By this technique, a blue dye- and a technetium-labeled colloid is injected at the site of the primary tumor or primary tumor resection scar. The agents are taken up by the locoregional lymphatic drainage system with areas of sentinel lymph node(s) identified by gamma scan and then individual nodes can be identified by their uptake of blue dye [63–65]. Selective excisional biopsies of these nodes can then be performed, with some having argued that if these nodes are negative there may be no need to proceed with a radical groin dissection.

In 2005, Kroon et al. [66] reported the 10 year of experience with DSNB at the Netherlands Cancer Institute (NCI). In 123 patients with clinically node-negative disease, 21% had a positive sentinel node. The 5-year disease-specific survival was 66% for those with a positive sentinel node and 96% for those with a negative sentinel node. The false-negative rate of this technique was, however, only 16%. Spiess et al. [67] investigated this method in 31 patients with invasive penile cancer and cN0 disease. All patients underwent a superficial inguinal lymph node dissection for full pathologic evaluation regardless of their sentinel node status. The reported sensitivity of DSNB in this study was only 71%, leading these authors to conclude that this technique was insufficient for detecting occult disease in cN0 patients.

Kroon et al. [66] suggested that one method to reduce the false-negative rate from DSNB is to first assess the nodes with ultrasound and FNA prior to DSNB. This method can potentially reduce not only the false-negative rate from DSNB but also the number of nodes requiring DSNB by identifying them first with FNA. Crawshaw et al. [35] assessed the use of dynamic lymphoscintigraphy combined with ultrasound-guided FNA in 66 patients with ≥ Stage T1, Grade 2 disease with clinically negative inguinal nodes. 17 patients (21 nodal groups) were found to have inguinal involvement by DSNB and ultrasound-guided FNA demonstrated metastases and eight nodal groups. In two patients who had an initially negative sentinel node biopsy, ultrasound suggested metastatic involvement and repeat biopsy confirmed micrometastatic disease. The remaining patients with negative DSNB did not demonstrate any evidence of disease at a range of follow-up between 6 and 28 months.

Leijte et al. [68] combined the NCI experience with that of the St. George's Hospital Group in London for a pooled study cohort of 323 patients. All patients underwent a preoperative ultrasound with possible FNA prior to DSNB. By this method, the combined false-negative rate at a median follow-up of 17.9 months was 7%. Although this false-negative rate remains of clinical concern in delaying potentially curative early inguinal lymphadenectomy, these data do represent a significant improvement as compared to earlier reports. Leijte et al. [69] also demonstrated using a hybrid single-photon emission computed tomography (SPECT)/CT scanner that lymphatic rerouting by tumor blockage of lymphatic channels can occur and may be an explanation for some false negatives with DSNB in a subset of patients (Fig. 4.4). The authors suggest that the identification of this phenomenon supports the utilization of ultrasound and FNA as adjunctive tools to DSNB.

Staging of Distant Metastases

Distant metastases in penile cancer typically occur late in the natural history of the disease, portending a poor prognosis, and are found in <2% of all cases at presentation [70]. The most common sites of distant metastasis are the liver, lung, and retroperitoneum [71].

Conventional Imaging and Standard Practice

Current standard practice is to investigate for distant metastatic disease using CT of the abdomen and pelvis and chest radiography. Imaging for the detection of distant metastases should be performed in the setting of palpable inguinal adenopathy, pathologic evidence of inguinal nodal involvement, or pathologic high-risk features of the primary tumor (corporal invasion, poorly differentiated primary tumor, LVI). A bone scan should be performed only in symptomatic patients or in the clinical context of an elevated alkaline phosphatase or serum calcium level, and in some cases of advanced disease.

PET–CT
While PET–CT has been helpful in some malignancies for the detection of distant metastatic disease, this has not been thoroughly investigated in penile cancer. As discussed above, Graafland et al. [52] investigated the use of PET–CT in

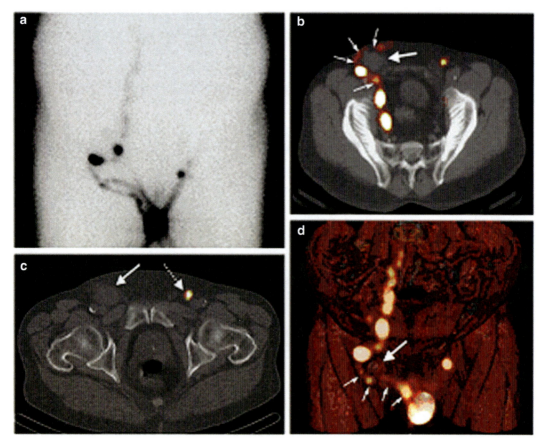

Fig. 4.4 SPECT/CT images demonstrate lymphatic rerouting around large metastatic lymph node in a 74-year-old penile cancer patient. (**a**) Conventional image demonstrates lymphatic drainage to both inguinal regions. (**c**) Fused SPECT/CT image demonstrates large right groin node with no uptake (*solid arrow*) but also shows sentinel node in left groin (*broken arrow*). (**b, d**). Fused SPECT/CT images (**b**: axial 2-dimensional; **d**: 3-dimensional) demonstrate lymphatic drainage being rerouted around large metastatic lymph node in right groin as well as uptake of tracer in pelvic nodes. Reprinted with permission of the Society of Nuclear Medicine from: Leijte JA, van der Ploeg IM, Valdes Olmos RA, Nieweg OE, Horenblas S. Visualization of tumor blockage and rerouting of lymphatic drainage in penile cancer patients by use of SPECT/CT. J Nucl Med. 2009 Mar;50(3):364–7, Fig. 1.

penile cancer, mainly for the purposes of regional lymph node imaging. The use of PET–CT in this study, however, did identify five patients with radiographic evidence of metastatic disease. These lesions were confirmed pathologically in four of these patients. Although this small subgroup analysis is inadequate to base management recommendations, it does indicate that this imaging modality may hold future promise for the assessment of distant metastases in select patients. Accurate detection of distant metastatic disease may help alter treatment algorithms, especially as effective systemic treatment regimens for advanced disease become readily available.

Conclusion

There are many aspects to the management of penile cancer in which imaging plays an important role. Accurate preoperative staging of the primary tumor can be very helpful in surgical planning and preparing patient expectations in regard to the ability for organ preservation versus the necessity for a more radical resection of the phallus. It is clear that MRI is the current preferred method for imaging the primary tumor. Although there are several imaging modalities under investigation for determining the presence of regional lymph node involvement, a truly accurate imaging technique has not yet emerged as the standard of care over surgical inguinal lymph node dissection. An improved method of imaging with an extremely low false-negative rate for nodal metastases in clinically node-negative patients would truly alter the treatment approach to this disease. While not currently adequate, it is hoped that one of these modalities under investigation will ultimately serve this need.

References

1. Edge SB, American Joint Committee on Cancer. AJCC cancer staging manual. 7th ed. New York: Springer; 2010.
2. Feldman AS, McDougal WS. Long-term outcome of excisional organ sparing surgery for carcinoma of the penis. J Urol. 2011;186(4):1303–7.
3. McDougal WS, Kirchner Jr FK, Edwards RH, Killion LT. Treatment of carcinoma of the penis: the case for primary lymphadenectomy. J Urol. 1986;136(1): 38–41.
4. Horenblas S, van Tinteren H, Delemarre JF, Moonen LM, Lustig V, van Waardenburg EW. Squamous cell carcinoma of the penis. III. Treatment of regional lymph nodes. J Urol. 1993;149(3):492–7.
5. McDougal WS. Carcinoma of the penis: improved survival by early regional lymphadenectomy based on the histological grade and depth of invasion of the primary lesion. J Urol. 1995;154(4):1364–6.
6. Slaton JW, Morgenstern N, Levy DA, Santos Jr MW, Tamboli P, Ro JY, et al. Tumor stage, vascular invasion and the percentage of poorly differentiated cancer: independent prognosticators for inguinal lymph node metastasis in penile squamous cancer. J Urol. 2001;165(4):1138–42.
7. Ficarra V, Zattoni F, Artibani W, Fandella A, Martignoni G, Novara G, et al. Nomogram predictive of pathological inguinal lymph node involvement in patients with squamous cell carcinoma of the penis. J Urol. 2006;175(5):1700–4. discussion 1704–5.
8. Guimaraes GC, Lopes A, Campos RS, Zequi Sde C, Leal ML, Carvalho AL, et al. Front pattern of invasion in squamous cell carcinoma of the penis: new prognostic factor for predicting risk of lymph node metastases. Urology. 2006;68(1):148–53.
9. Dai B, Ye DW, Kong YY, Yao XD, Zhang HL, Shen YJ. Predicting regional lymph node metastasis in chinese patients with penile squamous cell carcinoma: The role of histopathological classification, tumor stage and depth of invasion. J Urol. 2006;176(4 Pt 1):1431–5. discussion 1435.
10. Lopes A, Hidalgo GS, Kowalski LP, Torloni H, Rossi BM, Fonseca FP. Prognostic factors in carcinoma of the penis: Multivariate analysis of 145 patients treated with amputation and lymphadenectomy. J Urol. 1996;156(5):1637–42.
11. Pizzocaro G, Algaba F, Horenblas S, Solsona E, Tana S, Van Der Poel H, et al. EAU penile cancer guidelines 2009. Eur Urol. 2010;57(6):1002–12.
12. Lont AP, Besnard AP, Gallee MP, van Tinteren H, Horenblas S. A comparison of physical examination and imaging in determining the extent of primary penile carcinoma. BJU Int. 2003;91(6):493–5.
13. Petralia G, Villa G, Scardino E, Zoffoli E, Renne G, de Cobelli O, et al. Local staging of penile cancer using magnetic resonance imaging with pharmacologically induced penile erection. Radiol Med. 2008;113(4):517–28.
14. Raghavaiah NV. Corpus cavernosogram in the evaluation of carcinoma of the penis. J Urol. 1978;120(4): 423–4.
15. Escribano G, Allona A, Burgos FJ, Garcia R, Navio S, Escudero A. Cavernosography in diagnosis of metastatic tumors of the penis: 5 new cases and a review of the literature. J Urol. 1987;138(5):1174–7.
16. Haddad FS, Kovac A, Kivirand A, Sonkin B. Cavernosography in diagnosis of penile metastases secondary to bladder cancer. Urology. 1985;26(6): 585–6.
17. Bertolotto M, Serafini G, Dogliotti L, Gandolfo N, Gandolfo NG, Belgrano M, et al. Primary and secondary malignancies of the penis: ultrasound features. Abdom Imaging. 2005;30(1):108–12.
18. Horenblas S, Kroger R, Gallee MP, Newling DW, van Tinteren H. Ultrasound in squamous cell carcinoma of the penis; a useful addition to clinical staging? A comparison of ultrasound with histopathology. Urology. 1994;43(5):702–7.
19. Solsona E, Algaba F, Horenblas S, Pizzocaro G, Windahl T. European Association of Urology. EAU guidelines on penile cancer. Eur Urol. 2004;46(1): 1–8.
20. Stewart SB, Leder RA, Inman BA. Imaging tumors of the penis and urethra. Urol Clin North Am. 2010;37(3):353–67.
21. Kochhar R, Taylor B, Sangar V. Imaging in primary penile cancer: current status and future directions. Eur Radiol. 2010;20(1):36–47.
22. Fujita H. New horizons in MR technology: RF coil designs and trends. Magn Reson Med Sci. 2007;6(1): 29–42.
23. Scardino E, Villa G, Bonomo G, Matei DV, Verweij F, Rocco B, et al. Magnetic resonance imaging combined with artificial erection for local staging of penile cancer. Urology. 2004;63(6):1158–62.
24. Dewire D, Lepor H. Anatomic considerations of the penis and its lymphatic drainage. Urol Clin North Am. 1992;19(2):211–9.
25. Ravi R. Correlation between the extent of nodal involvement and survival following groin dissection for carcinoma of the penis. Br J Urol. 1993;72(5 Pt 2): 817–9.

26. Srinivas V, Morse MJ, Herr HW, Sogani PC, Whitmore Jr WF. Penile cancer: relation of extent of nodal metastasis to survival. J Urol. 1987;137(5):880–2.

27. Ornellas AA, Seixas AL, Marota A, Wisnescky A, Campos F, de Moraes JR. Surgical treatment of invasive squamous cell carcinoma of the penis: retrospective analysis of 350 cases. J Urol. 1994;151(5): 1244–9.

28. Theodorescu D, Russo P, Zhang ZF, Morash C, Fair WR. Outcomes of initial surveillance of invasive squamous cell carcinoma of the penis and negative nodes. J Urol. 1996;155(5):1626–31.

29. Hardner GJ, Bhanalaph T, Murphy GP, Albert DJ, Moore RH. Carcinoma of the penis: analysis of therapy in 100 consecutive cases. J Urol. 1972;108(3): 428–30.

30. Bhagat SK, Gopalakrishnan G, Kekre NS, Chacko NK, Kumar S, Manipadam MT, et al. Factors predicting inguinal node metastasis in squamous cell cancer of penis. World J Urol. 2010;28(1):93–8.

31. Spiess PE, Hernandez MS, Pettaway CA. Contemporary inguinal lymph node dissection: minimizing complications. World J Urol. 2009;27(2): 205–12.

32. Hughes B, Leijte J, Shabbir M, Watkin N, Horenblas S. Non-invasive and minimally invasive staging of regional lymph nodes in penile cancer. World J Urol. 2009;27(2):197–203.

33. Esen G. Ultrasound of superficial lymph nodes. Eur J Radiol. 2006;58(3):345–59.

34. Steinkamp HJ, Mueffelmann M, Bock JC, Thiel T, Kenzel P, Felix R. Differential diagnosis of lymph node lesions: a semiquantitative approach with colour doppler ultrasound. Br J Radiol. 1998;71(848): 828–33.

35. Crawshaw JW, Hadway P, Hoffland D, Bassingham S, Corbishley CM, Smith Y, et al. Sentinel lymph node biopsy using dynamic lymphoscintigraphy combined with ultrasound-guided fine needle aspiration in penile carcinoma. Br J Radiol. 2009;82(973):41–8.

36. Tabatabaei S, Harisinghani M, McDougal WS. Regional lymph node staging using lymphotropic nanoparticle enhanced magnetic resonance imaging with ferumoxtran-10 in patients with penile cancer. J Urol. 2005;174(3):923–7. discussion 927.

37. Graafland NM, Teertstra HJ, Besnard AP, van Boven HH, Horenblas S. Identification of high risk pathological node positive penile carcinoma: value of preoperative computerized tomography imaging. J Urol. 2011;185(3):881–7.

38. Jung CW, Jacobs P. Physical and chemical properties of superparamagnetic iron oxide MR contrast agents: ferumoxides, ferumoxtran, ferumoxsil. Magn Reson Imaging. 1995;13(5):661–74.

39. Weissleder R, Elizondo G, Wittenberg J, Lee AS, Josephson L, Brady TJ. Ultrasmall superparamagnetic iron oxide: an intravenous contrast agent for assessing lymph nodes with MR imaging. Radiology. 1990;175(2): 494–8.

40. Weissleder R, Elizondo G, Wittenberg J, Rabito CA, Bengele HH, Josephson L. Ultrasmall superparamagnetic iron oxide: characterization of a new class of contrast agents for MR imaging. Radiology. 1990; 175(2):489–93.

41. Guimaraes R, Clement O, Bittoun J, Carnot F, Frija G. MR lymphography with superparamagnetic iron nanoparticles in rats: pathologic basis for contrast enhancement. AJR Am J Roentgenol. 1994; 162(1):201–7.

42. Clement O, Guimaraes R, de Kerviler E, Frija G. Magnetic resonance lymphography. Enhancement patterns using superparamagnetic nanoparticles. Invest Radiol. 1994;29 Suppl 2:S226–S8.

43. Bellin MF, Lebleu L, Meric JB. Evaluation of retroperitoneal and pelvic lymph node metastases with MRI and MR lymphangiography. Abdom Imaging. 2003;28(2):155–63.

44. Harisinghani MG, Barentsz JO, Hahn PF, Deserno W, de la Rosette J, Saini S, et al. MR lymphangiography for detection of minimal nodal disease in patients with prostate cancer. Acad Radiol. 2002;9 Suppl 2:S312–S3.

45. Pannu HK, Wang KP, Borman TL, Bluemke DA. MR imaging of mediastinal lymph nodes: Evaluation using a superparamagnetic contrast agent. J Magn Reson Imaging. 2000;12(6):899–904.

46. Harisinghani MG, Barentsz J, Hahn PF, Deserno WM, Tabatabaei S, van de Kaa CH, et al. Noninvasive detection of clinically occult lymph-node metastases in prostate cancer. N Engl J Med. 2003;348(25): 2491–9.

47. Fletcher JW, Djulbegovic B, Soares HP, Siegel BA, Lowe VJ, Lyman GH, et al. Recommendations on the use of 18F-FDG PET in oncology. J Nucl Med. 2008;49(3):480–508.

48. Lardinois D, Weder W, Hany TF, Kamel EM, Korom S, Seifert B, et al. Staging of non-small-cell lung cancer with integrated positron-emission tomography and computed tomography. N Engl J Med. 2003; 348(25):2500–7.

49. Antoch G, Saoudi N, Kuehl H, Dahmen G, Mueller SP, Beyer T, et al. Accuracy of whole-body dual-modality fluorine-18-2-fluoro-2-deoxy-D-glucose positron emission tomography and computed tomography (FDG-PET/CT) for tumor staging in solid tumors: Comparison with CT and PET. J Clin Oncol. 2004;22(21):4357–68.

50. Ng SH, Yen TC, Chang JT, Chan SC, Ko SF, Wang HM, et al. Prospective study of [18F]fluorodeoxyglucose positron emission tomography and computed tomography and magnetic resonance imaging in oral cavity squamous cell carcinoma with palpably negative neck. J Clin Oncol. 2006;24(27):4371–6.

51. Scher B, Seitz M, Reiser M, Hungerhuber E, Hahn K, Tiling R, et al. 18F-FDG PET/CT for staging of penile cancer. J Nucl Med. 2005;46(9):1460–5.

52. Graafland NM, Leijte JA, Valdes Olmos RA, Hoefnagel CA, Teertstra HJ, Horenblas S. Scanning

with 18F-FDG-PET/CT for detection of pelvic nodal involvement in inguinal node-positive penile carcinoma. Eur Urol. 2009;56(2):339–45.

53. Leijte JA, Graafland NM, Valdes Olmos RA, van Boven HH, Hoefnagel CA, Horenblas S. Prospective evaluation of hybrid 18F-fluorodeoxyglucose positron emission tomography/computed tomography in staging clinically node-negative patients with penile carcinoma. BJU Int. 2009;104(5):640–4.

54. Souillac I, Rigaud J, Ansquer C, Marconnet L, Bouchot O. Prospective evaluation of (18) F-fluorodeoxyglucose positron emission tomography-computerized tomography to assess inguinal lymph node status in invasive squamous cell carcinoma of the penis. J Urol. 2012;187(2):493–7.

55. Sadeghi R, Gholami H, Zakavi SR, Kakhki VR, Horenblas S. Accuracy of 18F-FDG PET/CT for diagnosing inguinal lymph node involvement in penile squamous cell carcinoma: systematic review and meta-analysis of the literature. Clin Nucl Med. 2012;37(5):436–41.

56. Cabanas RM. An approach for the treatment of penile carcinoma. Cancer. 1977;39(2):456–66.

57. Cabanas RM. Anatomy and biopsy of sentinel lymph nodes. Urol Clin North Am. 1992;19(2):267–76.

58. Perinetti E, Crane DB, Catalona WJ. Unreliability of sentinel lymph node biopsy for staging penile carcinoma. J Urol. 1980;124(5):734–5.

59. Wespes E, Simon J, Schulman CC. Cabanas approach: is sentinel node biopsy reliable for staging penile carcinoma? Urology. 1986;28(4):278–9.

60. Srinivas V, Joshi A, Agarwal B, Mundhada U, Shah A, Phadke AG. Penile cancer—the sentinel lymph node controversy. Urol Int. 1991;47(2):108–9.

61. Pettaway CA, Pisters LL, Dinney CP, Jularbal F, Swanson DA, von Eschenbach AC, et al. Sentinel lymph node dissection for penile carcinoma: The M. D. Anderson Cancer Center experience. J Urol. 1995;154(6):1999–2003.

62. Morton DL, Wen DR, Wong JH, Economou JS, Cagle LA, Storm FK, et al. Technical details of intraoperative lymphatic mapping for early stage melanoma. Arch Surg. 1992;127(4):392–9.

63. Han KR, Brogle BN, Goydos J, Perrotti M, Cummings KB, Weiss RE. Lymphatic mapping and intraoperative lymphoscintigraphy for identifying the sentinel node in penile tumors. Urology. 2000;55(4):582–5.

64. Valdes Olmos RA, Tanis PJ, Hoefnagel CA, Jansen L, Nieweg OE, Meinhardt W, et al. Penile lymphoscintigraphy for sentinel node identification. Eur J Nucl Med. 2001;28(5):581–5.

65. Tanis PJ, Lont AP, Meinhardt W, Olmos RA, Nieweg OE, Horenblas S. Dynamic sentinel node biopsy for penile cancer: reliability of a staging technique. J Urol. 2002;168(1):76–80.

66. Kroon BK, Horenblas S, Meinhardt W, van der Poel HG, Bex A, van Tinteren H, et al. Dynamic sentinel node biopsy in penile carcinoma: evaluation of 10 years experience. Eur Urol. 2005;47(5):601–6. discussion 606.

67. Spiess PE, Izawa JI, Bassett R, Kedar D, Busby JE, Wong F, et al. Preoperative lymphoscintigraphy and dynamic sentinel node biopsy for staging penile cancer: results with pathological correlation. J Urol. 2007;177(6):2157–61.

68. Leijte JA, Hughes B, Graafland NM, Kroon BK, Olmos RA, Nieweg OE, et al. Two-center evaluation of dynamic sentinel node biopsy for squamous cell carcinoma of the penis. J Clin Oncol. 2009;27(20): 3325–9.

69. Leijte JA, van der Ploeg IM, Valdes Olmos RA, Nieweg OE, Horenblas S. Visualization of tumor blockage and rerouting of lymphatic drainage in penile cancer patients by use of SPECT/CT. J Nucl Med. 2009;50(3):364–7.

70. Rippentrop JM, Joslyn SA, Konety BR. Squamous cell carcinoma of the penis: evaluation of data from the surveillance, epidemiology, and end results program. Cancer. 2004;101(6):1357–63.

71. Singh AK, Saokar A, Hahn PF, Harisinghani MG. Imaging of penile neoplasms. Radiographics. 2005; 25(6):1629–38.

Penile-Sparing Approaches to Primary Penile Tumours

Hussain M. Alnajjar, Majid Shabbir, and
Nicholas A. Watkin

Introduction

An increase in the understanding of the natural history of penile cancer has lead to a paradigm shift in how this rare malignancy is treated. In the past, the tendency had been towards radical surgery with frequent overtreatment of the primary lesion. While such surgery achieved excellent oncological control, its emasculating consequences led to serious psychological and sexual morbidity [1]. Over the last decade, the surgical management of penile cancer has been revolutionised. Challenges to the traditional belief that a 2 cm margin was required for adequate clearance have paved the way to the concept of new surgical techniques that aim to minimise the impact of the disease and its treatment on the quality of life by preserving as much normal functional penile tissue as possible, without compromising oncological control. This is especially relevant when planning treatment in the cohort of men who develop the disease at a younger age (approximately 20% <40 year at presentation [2]).

Studies over the past decade have challenged the need for such extensive margins. Agrawal et al. reviewed 64 partial and total penectomy specimens, to determine the microscopic spread of tumour beyond the visible tumour margin [3]. They found only 19% of cases had microscopic extension beyond the gross tumour margin. Of these, 75% were ≤5 mm form the margin. Hoffman et al. reported on their experience of 14 patients who underwent conventional surgery for penile cancer [4]. Half the group had excision margins of ≤10 mm, although this had no bearing on recurrence as no patient in their series developed recurrences after 33 months follow-up. In a series looking at penile preserving techniques, approximately half of the 51 patients in the series had clear surgical margins of ≤10 mm, including 33% with margins ≤5 mm. Despite this, the local recurrence rate was only 4% after a mean follow-up of 26 months, confirming that comparable oncological control to conventional radical surgery could be achieved with excision margins of only a few millimetres [5].

As a result of these studies, there has been a move away from more radical surgery to a variety of penile preserving techniques. The use of these techniques has been more prevalent in Western countries such as the UK, where approximately 80% of malignant lesions present on the glans penis and prepuce and are more amenable to an organ conserving approach [6, 7]. Selection of the most appropriate technique is dependent on the stage and location of

H.M. Alnajjar, M.B.B.S., B.Sc. (Med Sci.), M.R.C.S.
M. Shabbir, F.R.C.S. (Urol) • N.A. Watkin, M.Ch.,
F.R.C.S. (Urol) (✉)
Department of Urology, St. George's Hospital,
Blackshaw Rd, London SW17 0QT, UK
e-mail: nick.watkin@stgeorges.nhs.uk

P.E. Spiess (ed.), *Penile Cancer: Diagnosis and Treatment*, Current Clinical Urology,
DOI 10.1007/978-1-62703-367-1_5, © Springer Science+Business Media New York 2013

the primary tumour and the various options are discussed further below. Treatment is tailored to the individual, taking into account the lesion, the effect of surgery on penile length, the patient's age and co-morbidities. Knowledge and expertise with the different surgical techniques is vital to ensure the best cosmetic, functional, psychological and oncological outcome in patients who present with this potentially devastating disease. Here, we discuss the different treatment modalities available and their role in the management of penile cancer.

Topical Therapies

Suitable for Stage Tis Disease Only

The non-invasive nature of carcinoma in situ (Tis) of the penis makes it amenable to a number of different treatments. Topical application of 5% 5-Fluorouracil (5-FU) chemotherapeutic agent is the most commonly used first line treatment. It is best suited to immunocompetent patients with small (1–2 cm), mucosal and superficial lesions. It has poor efficacy in the immunosuppressed or those with widespread "field changes" [8]. It is usually applied topically for 4 weeks on alternate days, and is safe, with low morbidity and minimal systemic absorption. The largest study to date reported overall response rates with 5-FU of 50% at 3 years [9].

Non- or partial responders are usually treated with immunotherapy using 5% imiquimod (IQ) cream for a similar length of time and regimen as second line treatment [10]. Although the exact mechanism of action of this novel immunomodulatory therapy is unclear, it is believed to activate the patient's host immune system leading to secretion of cytokines such as interferon-α, tumour necrosis factor and various interleukins (IFNα, IL-1, 6, 12, TNFα). While success has been reported in a number of case reports and small case series, no large-scale long-term efficacy data is currently available [8, 10]. The overall response rate to topical agents has been reported to be approximately 57% [9].

Laser Therapy

Best Suited to Stage Tis, But Has Been Used up to Stage T2 Lesions

Lasers have been used to treat a range of penile lesions from stage Tis to larger T2 lesions. Two types have been used; The carbon dioxide (CO_2) laser and the neodymium:yttrium aluminium garnet (Nd:YAG) laser.

The CO_2 laser has a tissue penetration of 2–2.5 mm and has the advantage of also being able to be used as a scalpel to excise tissue for histological analysis by direct focussing of the beam. Ablations sites generally heal in 3–4 weeks. The Nd:YAG laser has a tissue penetration of 3–5 mm allowing treatment of more invasive lesions, but it causes tissue coagulation preventing histological diagnosis, and a risk of understaging the disease. Ablation sites can take up to 2–3 months to heal. Treatment with either of these lasers is usually well tolerated, with good cosmetic and functional results. Minor complications ranging from minor pain and bleeding at treatment sites, to preputial lymphoedema in those patients who have retained their foreskin have been reported [11]. However, despite its potential, this technique has not been as widely adopted as expected, largely due to the high re-treatment and progression rate, which is reportedly proportional to the stage being treated. In one study consisting of 19 patients with Tis treated with laser therapy, 26% of patients required re-treatment for a histologically confirmed Tis recurrence at a mean follow-up of 32 months, while 1 patient (5%) progressed to invasive disease [12]. In another study assessing the combined use of both lasers, 13 of 67 patients (19%) had disease recurrence, with upgrading from the original tumour in 3 of 13 (23%) cases [13]. The recurrence rate for Tis was 14%, and 21% for stage T1–T2 disease. A disease progression rate of 5% (nodal disease) was also reported. More recent studies treating a greater number of T1–T2 lesions reported a higher overall recurrence, and nodal progression rate (48% and

Table 5.1 Oncological outcomes following laser therapy

Study	Patients (T stage)	Reported outcomes	Mean follow-up (months)	Treatment
Van Bezooijen et al. [12]	19 (Tis)	Local relapse 26% Progression rate 5%	32	CO_2 and Nd:YAG
Windahl et al. [13]	21 (Tis) 56 (T1–T2)	Local relapse 14.2% (Tis) 21.7% (T1–T2) Overall progression rate 5%	42	CO_2 and Nd:YAG
Meijer et al. [14]	6 (Tis) 38 (T1–T2)	Local relapse Overall 48% Progression rate 23%	44	Nd:YAG
Schlenker et al. [30]	11 (Tis) 43 (T1–T2)	Local relapse overall 42% No progression reported	87	Nd:YAG

T tumour stage, *Tis* carcinoma in-situ, CO_2 carbon dioxide, *Nd:YAG* neodymium:yttrium aluminium garnet laser

23%, respectively) [14], highlighting the inadequacy of laser treatment for invasive disease (Table 5.1).

Penile-Sparing Surgical Techniques

Surgery has an important and evolving role in the treatment of penile CIS.

Circumcision: Suitable for Any Lesion Confined Solely to the Prepuce

Circumcision plays a key role in the management of penile cancer. It not only removes any lesion confined solely to the prepuce, but is also of benefit in cases of glanular Tis where it prevents the persistence of a micro-environment suited to HPV infection as well as chronic inflammation and progression to invasive disease. Circumcision also aides the management of Tis by facilitating clinical examination at follow-up, and allowing easier application and retention of topical therapies, as well as preventing the development of preputial oedema associated with laser therapy. Removal of the foreskin is therefore of great benefit in patients with penile cancer.

When performing the circumcision, it is essential to obtain an adequate clearance margin and exclude concurrent glanular disease. In difficult cases, a swab soaked in 5% acetic acid applied to the penis for up to 5 min has been used to help detect occult areas of Tis, staining the abnormal areas white ("acetowhite" reaction), to help guide the extent of excision [6, 9]. However, the use of visual inspection after acetic acid staining has been discredited by many due to its poor sensitivity for detecting the HPV component of Tis (50%) in addition to high false positive staining [15–17].

Total Glans Resurfacing: Suitable for Glanular Tis/Ta, and up to Stage T1a Disease

Surgical excision of Tis affecting the glans penis has been advocated for patients who have extensive field change, in those unlikely or unwilling to adhere to strict treatment and surveillance protocols, and those with recurrent disease or failure of other conservative therapies. Repeated topical therapies can cause scarring and an unsightly appearance of glans which can make monitoring for recurrence difficult.

Total glans resurfacing (TGR) is the best surgical approach to treatment, excising the diseased area with an adequate margin followed by extra-genital split thickness skin graft. This technique was first described by Bracka for the management of severe *Balanitis Xerotica Obilterans* (BXO), but has been adapted for Tis/Ta disease [18, 19].

The procedure is performed under a general anaesthetic with preoperative antibiotic coverage and with the use of a penile tourniquet. The glans epithelium is marked in quadrants from the meatus to the coronal sulcus. A perimeatal and

Table 5.2 Oncological outcomes following glans resurfacing

Study	Patients (T stage)	Reported outcomes	Mean follow-up (months)	Treatment	Comments
Hadway et al. [19]	10 (Tis)	No recurrence/ progression	30	TGR	All refractory to topical agents or progressed to extensive disease
Shabbir et al. [20]	25 (Tis)	Recurrence 4%, no progression	29	TGR/PGR	Unexpected invasive disease 40% Early revision rate 28% (20% for invasive disease, 8% PSM)
Ayres et al. [21]	36 (T1aG2)	Early revision rate 8% Local recurrence rate 6%	21	TGR	Unexpected invasive disease in 17% (pre-op biopsy CIS only)
Shabbir et al. [20]	7 (T1aG2)	No recurrence or progression	29	TGR (5) PGR (2)	

Tis/CIS carcinoma in-situ, *T* tumour stage, *G* tumour grade, *TGR* total glans resurfacing, *PGR* partial glans resurfacing, *PSM* positive surgical margin

circumferential coronal incision is performed, and the glans epithelium and sub-epithelial tissue is then excised from the underlying spongiosum, starting from the meatus to the coronal sulcus for each respective quadrant. Deep spongiosal biopsies can be taken from each quadrant for separate pathological analysis and exclusion of invasion. An extra-genital split thickness skin graft, harvested from the thigh with an air dermatome, is used to cover the denuded glans. Graft thickness can range from 0.008 to 0.016 in. The graft is sutured and quilted using multiple 5-0 interrupted vicryl sutures. The patient is then catheterised (using a 14 French silicone catheter) and the glans penis is dressed with soft paraffin gauze followed by foam dressing to help protect and immobilise the graft. The dressing is left in place for 5 days with the patient remaining on strict bed rest for the first 48 h. On the fifth day, the dressing and catheter are removed, and the patient is discharged with wound care reassessment in clinic the following week. This approach allows preservation of maximal penile length, form and function and combines safe oncological control with a good cosmetic appearance. In a series of ten patients treated with TGR for recurrent, refractory or extensive disease, no patient had evidence of disease recurrence after a mean follow-up of 30 months. In addition, over 80% were sexually active within 3 months of surgery [19].

One of the main advantages of this minimally invasive surgical approach is its combined diagnostic and therapeutic ability. Whilst completely removing the diseased epithelium, total surgical excision also allows more accurate histopathological staging and diagnosis than the smaller incisional biopsies used with less invasive topical therapies. In a recent series assessing the use of glans resurfacing for Tis as a primary therapy, 10 of 25 patients (40%) had evidence of invasive carcinoma on the final pathological specimens despite all 25 patients having had preoperative incisional biopsies confirming evidence of Tis only [20]. This is alarming, given the fact that most patients diagnosed with Tis of the glans are primarily treated on the basis of incisional biopsies alone, and are thereafter usually treated with topical chemotherapy or laser as a first line treatment modality, which would not address any invasive component of the tumour adequately. This fact may as well explain the higher recurrence rate with laser therapy (26%), compared to surgical excision/resection (0–4%) [13, 19, 20]. These findings would support the primary use of surgery to avoid the risk of understaging, inadequate treatment and subsequent cancer progression (Table 5.2). It may also lead to a paradigm shift in our approach to managing glanular Tis in the future.

TGR can also be used to treat stage T1a disease. The procedure is no different to that used for non-invasive lesions, and is effective for T1a disease as the technique involves complete removal of the glans epithelium and sub-epithelial layers.

In a series assessing outcome of TGR for glanular CIS, seven patients were found to have unexpected foci of pT1G2 disease which was fully excised. No recurrences have been seen in this subset at a mean follow-up of 29 months [20]. Ayres et al. reported in a series of 36 patients, a positive margin rate of 11% and a revision rate of 8% following TGR for low/intermediate grade squamous cell carcinoma (SCC). Six men (17%) had invasive disease diagnosed unexpectedly following TGR for biopsy proven pre-malignant lesions [21].

Partial Glans Resurfacing: Suitable for Isolated Foci of Tis/Ta Affecting <50% of the Glans

Partial glans resurfacing (PGR) has also been used as a primary surgical approach for the treatment of localised glanular Tis that has failed to respond to conservative management. This technique involves the same principles as TGR, but is used in cases of solitary, localised foci of Tis affecting <50% of the glans. This approach has the advantage of conserving normal glans skin, allowing better preservation of glanular sensation, and achieving a final appearance similar to the original glans. This approach would be more attractive to younger, sexually active men. In a reported series of primary partial and TGR, PGR was associated with a very high risk of positive surgical margins (67%). Forty percent of this group required further surgical intervention, of which 13% was for positive Tis at the margin and 26% was due to unexpected invasive disease in the final specimen. Patients were still amenable to further penile preserving techniques, including TGR and glansectomy.

Despite the higher positive margin rate and need for further surgery, the PGR subgroup still had no cases of recurrence or progression at a mean follow-up of 29 months [20]. While the exact role and position of PGR in the management of Tis remains unclear, this technique may have a limited role in the management of glanular Tis in carefully selected cases.

Moh's Micrographic Surgery: Most Suitable for Stage T1a, But Has Been Used up to Stage T3

An alternative surgical approach is excision using Moh's micrographic surgery (MMS). This technique involves removing the entire lesion in thin sections, with concurrent histological examination to ensure clear margins microscopically [22]. This technique allows maximal preservation of normal penile tissue, but is difficult and time consuming, requiring both a surgeon and pathologist trained in this technique to ensure adequate oncological clearance. Despite maximal length preservation, the final cosmetic result from this procedure can be quite poor. A recent review of outcome from this technique reported a high (32%) recurrence rate [23], and the uptake and use of the technique worldwide has been very limited.

Wide Local Excision/Partial Glansectomy: Suitable for Small, Discrete Lesions on the Glans up to Stage T1a

Small, discrete lesions on the glans can be treated by wide local excision, or partial glansectomy. If the defect after excision is small, and not too close to the urethral meatus, primary closure can be achieved with only minimal glans deformity. Larger defects may be difficult to close without tilting the glans and causing problems directing micturition. In such cases, a split skin graft may be required to cover the defect and improve the final cosmetic appearance and functional outcome.

Penile preserving techniques such as partial glansectomy and TGR are best suited to patients with "low risk" T1a disease (well moderately differentiated G1/G2 disease, with no evidence of lymphovascular invasion). Close surveillance and follow-up is essential to ensure early detection of any recurrences. Careful patient selection is vital, and these techniques should only be offered to those well motivated and compliant to ensure close surveillance and success form this surgical approach. Local recurrence, or positive surgical margins, should be treated by total glansectomy, and early detection with subsequent "salvage" surgery has a high success rate, with no adverse impact on disease specific survival [24, 25]. Patients with "high risk" T1b disease (poorly or undifferentiated G3 disease, or with evidence of lymphovascular invasion) are best managed by glansectomy at the outset and this technique is described in detail below.

Glansectomy and Reconstruction: Suitable for Stage T1b/T2 Tumours Confined to the Glans

The management of T2 lesions confined to the glans has benefited greatly from developments in penile preserving techniques. Glansectomy is the best surgical approach for T2 disease affecting the corpus spongiosum, and high risk T1b disease. This procedure utilises knowledge of the anatomical planes between the corpora cavernosa and corpus spongiosum first described by Austoni et al. [26]. In this procedure, the glans penis is dissected from the corpora cavernosa, with the subsequent formation of a new urethral meatus at the tip of the shaft. The procedure can be combined with a split thickness skin graft to create a "neo-glans" with excellent cosmesis and a near normal appearance, or can employ an advancement flap of shaft skin to cover the corporal tips and maintain a functional penis, albeit with a less satisfactory cosmetic appearance.

The procedure is performed under a general anaesthetic with preoperative antibiotic coverage and with the use of a tourniquet. A circumferential incision is made a centimetre below the corona on the distal shaft toward Buck's fascia. A plane of dissection is then created either above the dartos fascia, or below Buck's fascia, depending on the depth and extent of the glanular lesion. The glans "cap" is dissected free of the corporal heads, taking care not to stray into the spongiosum. Frozen sections from the corporal tips and distal urethral can be taken intra-operatively to ensure adequate surgical margins if any clinical doubt exists. In cases where the frozen section yields a positive margin, further "shaving" of the

corporal tips or urethra can be performed prior to any planned reconstruction.

As part of the reconstruction, the urethra is spatulated and can also be mobilised, if its position is too ventral, to a more central location at the tip of the penis. The shaft skin is then secured 2–3 cm from the tip of the penis using multiple 4-0 interrupted vicryl sutures. A split thickness skin graft, harvested from the thigh with an air dermatome, is used to cover the "exposed" glans. Graft thickness can range from 0.008 to 0.016 in. The graft is sutured and quilted using multiple 5-0 interrupted vicryl sutures. The patient is then catheterised (using a 14 French silicone catheter) and the glans penis is dressed with a soft paraffin dressing and gauze followed by foam dressing to help immobilise the graft. The dressing is left in place for 5 days with the patient remaining on strict bed rest for the first 48 h. On the fifth day, the dressing and catheter can be removed if the graft has taken well, followed by which the patient is discharged with wound care advice for review in clinic the following week. This approach allows maximal preservation of penile length, form and function, while combining good oncological results with an excellent cosmetic appearance.

Hatzichristou et al. reported seven cases of verrucous carcinomas treated by glansectomy without reconstruction [27]. Only one patient required further surgery due to local recurrence at 3 months. All patients returned to normal sexual function 1 month post-operatively and all are alive and disease free at 18–65 months follow-up. Morelli et al. reported their experience with glansectomy and reconstruction in 15 patients with SCC confined to the glans. At a mean follow-up of 36 months, all patients were disease free, with no cases of local recurrence. All were fully sexually active 2–6 months post-operatively, and while all had reduced neo-glans sensitivity, all had preserved orgasm and ejaculatory function highlighting the excellent functional preservation seen with this surgical approach [28]. In the largest reported series to date, only three local recurrences were seen in 72 patients treated by glansectomy and reconstruction at a mean follow-up of 27 months [29]. The recurrence rate of 4% is similar to that reported from more radical

Table 5.3 Oncological outcomes following glansectomy

Study	Procedure	Patients (number)	Local recurrence rate (%)	Mean follow-up (months)
Pietrzak et al. [6]	Partial/total glansectomy	39	2.5	16
Brown et al. [7]	Partial/total glansectomy	5	0	12
Gulino et al. [31]	Partial/total glansectomy	14	0	13
Smith et al. [29]	Partial/total glansectomy	72	4	27
Palminteri et al. [32]	Partial/total glansectomy	12	0	32
Morelli et al. [28]	Partial/total glansectomy	15	0	36
O'Kane et al. [33]	Total glansectomy	25	4	28

Table 5.4 Oncological outcomes following partial penectomy

Study	Patients (number)	Local recurrence rate (%)	Mean follow-up (months)
Bañón et al. [34]	42	7.1	67
Ficarra et al. [35]	30	0	69
Rempelakos et al. [36]	227	0	>120
Chen et al. [37]	34	5.8	37
Korets et al. [38]	32	3.2	34
Leijte et al. [39]	214	5.3	60.6
Ornellas et al. [40]	522	4	11

partial penectomy series, highlighting the comparable oncological outcomes using this more penile preserving approach (Table 5.3).

Distal Corporectomy/Partial Penectomy and Reconstruction: Suitable for Stage T2b/Distal T3 Disease

Evidence of disease extension into the corporeal bodies or urethra requires more extensive resection. The surgical procedure needs to be tailored to the site and size of the lesion, taking into account the overall penile length. The mainstay of treatment for tumours extending into corporal bodies or urethra is partial penectomy, although as resection margins of 2 cm maybe not required for a distal corporectomy. Partial penectomy has a low recurrence rate of 0–7% (Table 5.4). Excision should be combined with frozen section to ensure clear margins are achieved. Subsequent reconstructive techniques can be used to achieve a good cosmetic appearance. If the resultant phallus post-resection is too short, lengthening procedures can be used to allow the patient to stand to void, or have penetrative sex. In certain cases

where the disease is very proximal, or the resultant phallus too short, a subtotal or total penectomy and perineal urethrostomy may be more appropriate to achieve a better functional result.

The procedure is performed under a general anaesthetic with preoperative antibiotic coverage and with the use of a tourniquet. A circumferential incision is made 1–2 cm below the proximal limit of the tumour. The penile shaft skin is degloved to expose the underlying corpora. The corpora are incised to generate a "fish-mouth" appearance that will allow a vertical closure in the midline. A safe margin of 0.5–1 cm is considered for partial penectomy [5]. The urethra is divided to leave an additional length of approximately 1 cm from the end of the corporal dissection to allow for subsequent spatulation and reconstruction. Sections of the distal corporal margins and urethra are sent for frozen section to ensure adequate clearance. The corpora are closed using an absorbable 2-0 PDS suture. The overlying superficial dartos layer can then be reconstructed over the tips of the closed corpora, creating an excellent bed for the subsequent skin graft. As part of the reconstruction, the urethra is spatulated and can also be mobilised, if its position is too ventral, to a more central location at the tip of the penis. The shaft skin is then secured 2–3 cm from the tip of the penis using multiple 4-0 interrupted vicryl sutures. A split thickness skin graft, harvested from the thigh with an air dermatome, is used to cover the "exposed" glans. Graft thickness can range from 0.008 to 0.016 in. The graft is sutured and quilted using multiple 5-0 interrupted vicryl sutures. The patient is then catheterised (using a 14 French silicone catheter) and the glans penis is dressed with a soft paraffin dressing and gauze followed by foam dressing to help protect and immobilise the graft. The dressing is left in place for 5 days with the patient remaining on strict bed rest for the first 48 h. On the fifth day the dressing and catheter may be removed if the graft has taken adequately, and the patient is discharged with wound care advice for review in clinic the following week.

In cases where reconstruction using skin graft is not used or appropriate, shaft skin advancement flaps can be used to cover the corpora and meet the spatulated urethra. This approach often suits older patients who are medically unfit, or not keen for reconstruction. It may also be more suited to patients where cosmesis or sexual function is less important, although it is still possible to have erections and intercourse following this type of surgery. It has a significantly shorter operative time, and less need for restrictive bed rest, or skin graft care, hence constituting a good option in a select subset of patients.

Conclusion

Our knowledge of penile cancer and its treatment has advanced greatly over the last decade. The advent and development of new penile preserving treatments have achieved a better balance between excellent, reliable oncological control and a good cosmetic and functional result. It has substantially reduced the impact of the disease and its treatment on the majority of patients presenting with amenable lesions. Treatment in specialised centres well versed with the full range of different reconstructive techniques ensures the best outcome.

References

1. Opjordsmoen S, Fossa SD. Quality of life in patients treated for penile cancer. A follow-up study. Br J Urol. 1994;74(5):652–7.
2. Cancer trends in England and Wales, 1950–1999. www.statistics.gov.uk. Accessed 2004.
3. Agrawal A, Pai D, Ananthakrishnan N, et al. The histological extent of the local spread of carcinoma of the penis and its therapeutic implications. BJU Int. 2000;85(2):299–301.
4. Hoffman M, Renshaw A, Loughlin KR. Squamous cell carcinoma of the penis and microscopic pathologic margins. How much margin is needed for local cure? Cancer. 1999;85(7):1565–8.
5. Minhas S, Kayes O, Hegarty P, et al. What surgical resection margins are required to achieve oncological control in men with primary penile cancer? BJU Int. 2005;96:1040–3.
6. Pietrzak P, Corbishley C, Watkin N. Organ-sparing surgery for invasive penile cancer: early follow-up data. BJU Int. 2004;94(9):1253–7.
7. Brown CT, Minhas S, Ralph DJ. Conservative surgery for penile cancer: subtotal glans excision without grafting. BJU Int. 2005;96(6):911–2.
8. Porter WM, Francis N, Hawkins D, et al. Penile intraepithelial neoplasia: clinical spectrum and treatment of 35 cases. Br J Dermatol. 2002;147(6):1159–65.
9. Alnajjar HM, Lam W, Bolgeri M, Rees RW, Perry MJ, Watkin NA. Treatment of carcinoma in situ of the glans penis with topical chemotherapy agents. Eur Urol. 2012;62(5):923–8.
10. Micali G, Nasca MR, Tedeschi A. Topical treatment of intraepithelial penile carcinoma with imiquimod. Clin Exp Dermatol. 2003;28 Suppl 1:4–6.
11. Tietjen DN, Malek RS. Laser therapy of squamous cell dysplasia and carcinoma of the penis. Urology. 1998;52:559–65.
12. van Bezooijen BP, Horenblas S, Meinhardt W, Newling DW. Laser therapy for carcinoma in situ of the penis. J Urol. 2001;166(5):1670–1.
13. Windahl T, Andersson SO. Combined laser treatment for penile carcinoma: results after long-term follow up. J Urol. 2003;169(6):2118–21.
14. Meijer RP, Boon TA, van Venrooij GE, Wijburg CJ. Longterm follow-up after laser therapy for penile carcinoma. Urology. 2007;69(4):759–62.
15. Ekalaksananan T, Pientong C, Thinkhamrop J, Kongyingyoes B, Evans MF, Chaiwongkot A. Cervical cancer screening in north east Thailand using the visual inspection with acetic acid (VIA) test and its relationship to high-risk human papillomavirus (HR-HPV) status. J Obstet Gynaecol Res. 2010; 36(5):1037–43.
16. Kellokoski J, Syrjänen S, Kataja V, Yliskoski M, Syrjänen K. Acetowhite staining and its significance in diagnosis of oral mucosal lesions in women with genital HPV infections. J Oral Pathol Med. 1990; 19(6):278–83.

17. Frega A, French D, Pace S, Maranghi L, Palazzo A, Iacovelli R, et al. Prevalence of acetowhite areas in male partners of women affected by HPV and squamous intra-epithelial lesions (SIL) and their prognostic significance. A multicenter study. Anticancer Res. 2006;26(4B):3171–4.
18. Depasquale I, Park AJ, Bracka A. The treatment of balanitis xerotica obliterans. BJU Int. 2000;86: 459–65.
19. Hadway P, Corbishley CM, Watkin NA. Total glans resurfacing for premalignant lesions of the penis: initial outcome data. BJU Int. 2006;98(3):532–6.
20. Shabbir M, Muneer A, Kalsi J, Shukla CJ, Zacharakis E, Garaffa G, et al. Glans resurfacing for the treatment for carcinoma in situ of the penis: surgical technique and outcomes. Eur Urol. 2011;59(1):142–7.
21. Ayres B, Lam W, Al-Najjar H, Corbishley CM, Perry MJA, Watkin NA. Oncological outcomes of glans resurfacing in the treatment of selected superficially invasive penile cancers. J Urol. 2012;187(4): e306.
22. Mohs FE, Snow SN, Larson PO. Mohs micrographic surgery for penile tumors. Urol Clin North Am. 1992;19(2):291–304.
23. Shindel AW, Mann MW, Lev RY, Sengelmann R, Petersen J, Hruza GJ, et al. Mohs micrographic surgery for penile cancer: management and long-term followup. J Urol. 2007;178(5):1980–5.
24. Lindegaard JC, Nielsen OS, Lundbeck FA, et al. A retrospective analysis of 82 cases of cancer of the penis. BJU Int. 1996;77(6):883–90.
25. Lont AP, Gallee MPW, Meinhardt W, van Tinteren H, Horenblas S. Penis conserving treatment for T1 and T2 penile carcinoma: clinical implications of a local recurrence. J Urol. 2006;176(2):575–80.
26. Austoni E, Fenice O, Kartalas Goumas Y, et al. New trends in the surgical treatment of penile carcinoma. Arch Ital Urol Androl. 1996;68:163–8.
27. Hatzichristou DG, Apostolidis A, Tzortzis V, et al. Glansectomy: an alternative surgical treatment for Buschke-Lowenstein tumours of the penis. Urology. 2001;57:966–9.
28. Morelli G, Pagni R, Mariani C, Campo G, Menchini-Fabris F, Minervini R, et al. Glansectomy with split-thickness skin graft for the treatment of penile carcinoma. Int J Impot Res. 2009;21(5):311–4.
29. Smith Y, Hadway P, Biedrzycki O, et al. Reconstructive surgery for invasive squamous carcinoma of the glans penis. Eur Urol. 2007;52(4):1179–85.
30. Schlenker B, Gratzke C, Seitz M, Bader MJ, Reich O, Schneede P, et al. Fluorescence-guided laser therapy for penile carcinoma and precancerous lesions: long-term follow-up. Urol Oncol. 2011;29(6):788–93.
31. Gulino G, Sasso F, Falabella R, Bassi PF. Distal urethral reconstruction of the glans for penile carcinoma: results of a novel technique at 1-year of followup. J Urol. 2007;178(3 Pt 1):941–4.
32. Palminteri E, Berdondini E, Lazzeri M, Mirri F, Barbagli G. Resurfacing and reconstruction of the glans penis. Eur Urol. 2007;52(3):893–8.
33. O'Kane HF, Pahuja A, Ho KJ, Thwaini A, Nambirajan T, Keane P. Outcome of glansectomy and skin grafting in the management of penile cancer. Adv Urol. 2011;2011:240824.
34. Bañón Perez VJ, Nicolás Torralba JA, Valdelvira Nadal P, et al. [Squamous carcinoma of the penis] Carcinoma escamoso de pene. Arch Esp Urol. 2000; 53(8):693–9.
35. Ficarra V, Maffei N, Piacentini I, et al. Local treatment of penile squamous cell carcinoma. Urol Int. 2002;69(3):169–73.
36. Rempelakos A, Bastas E, Lymperakis CH, Thanos A. Carcinoma of the penis: experience from 360 cases. J BUON. 2004;9(1):51–5.
37. Chen MF, Chen WC, Wu CT, et al. Contemporary management of penile cancer including surgery and adjuvant radiotherapy: an experience in Taiwan. World J Urol. 2004;22(1):60–6.
38. Korets R, Koppie TM, Snyder ME, et al. Partial penectomy for patients with squamous cell carcinoma of the penis: the Memorial Sloan-Kettering experience. Ann Surg Oncol. 2007;14(12):3614–9.
39. Leijte JA, Kirrander P, Antonini N, et al. Recurrence patterns of squamous cell carcinoma of the penis: recommendations for follow up based on a two-centre analysis of 700 patients. Eur Urol. 2008;54(1): 161–8.
40. Ornellas AA, Kinchin EW, Nóbrega BL, Wisnescky A, Koifman N, Quirino R. Surgical treatment of invasive squamous cell carcinoma of the penis: Brazilian National Cancer Institute long-term experience. J Surg Oncol. 2008;97(6):487–95.

Surgical Concepts and Considerations of Inguinal Lymph Node Dissection for Penile Cancer

Cesar E. Ercole and Philippe E. Spiess

Introduction

Penile cancer is frequently (95%) of squamous cell carcinoma (SCC) histology and can impart disfiguring, mutilating, and severe consequences, especially when there is a delay in detection and treatment. Diagnosis of a primary penile tumor is based on clinical examination and a confirmatory tissue biopsy. Part of the difficulty in treating this lymphophilic tumor is the evaluation and treatment of the inguinal lymph nodes (ILN) which constitute the first echelon of regional metastatic progression in an often predictable pattern. A high degree of suspicion based on the clinical/pathologic features of the primary penile tumor and a thorough physical exam are paramount to the early detection of metastases to the ILN and especially since it can be surgically managed with curative intent. Early detection relies on the ability to perform a good physical exam; if this is not feasible (secondary to patient body habitus, prior surgical or radiation therapy), then other diagnostic modalities may be needed to ascertain the extent of disease and the potential for lymph

node involvement. Approximately 20–25% of patients who are clinically node negative (cN0) harbor occult metastatic disease [1]. It is imperative to note as well that the most important prognostic factor determining long-term survival in men with invasive penile SCC is the presence and extent of ILN involvement with early surgical intervention showing a strong impact on survival [2–8]. Careful consideration should be given if the patient presents with bulky nodal metastasis (>3 cm) and/or other sites of metastases, as these patients may most likely benefit from upfront systemic chemotherapy. Over the course of history, inguinal lymph node dissection (ILND) has been feared by patient and physician alike due to their historically high reported perioperative morbidity [4, 5]. Building on the pioneering work of many authors, the morbidity and surgical outcomes of ILND have been optimized integrating important concepts and considerations highlighted in the present chapter.

Penile Lymphatic System

The surgical planning of ILND requires proper knowledge of the penile/inguinal lymphatic anatomy and patterns of drainage. The lymphatic channels in large part follow the pattern of penile venous drainage. Traditionally, the lymphatics draining the penis have been grouped into a superficial and a deep group separated from one another via the fascia lata. Within the superficial group, there may be up to 25 lymph nodes situated

C.E. Ercole, M.D.
Department of Urology, University of South Florida, Tampa, FL, USA

P.E. Spiess, M.D., M.S. (✉)
Department of Genitourinary Oncology, Moffitt Cancer Center, 12902 Magnolia Drive, Office 12538, Tampa, FL 33612, USA
e-mail: philippe.spiess@moffitt.org

P.E. Spiess (ed.), *Penile Cancer: Diagnosis and Treatment*, Current Clinical Urology, DOI 10.1007/978-1-62703-367-1_6, © Springer Science+Business Media New York 2013 between Scarpa's fascia and the fascia lata. The superficial nodes may be further characterized based on their location into five zones by drawing a horizontal and vertical line through the point where the saphenous vein drains into the femoral vein. These five lymphatic zones comprise the superomedial, superolateral, inferomedial, inferolateral, and central lymph nodes, with the most common frequent site of metastasis being the superomedial area [9–14]. As the name of the deep inguinal nodes would imply, these lymph nodes are found below the fascia lata and medial to the femoral vein, with up to five nodes found in this area with the node of Cloquet being the most consistent lymph node within the femoral canal. Consideration needs to be given to the fact that there is crossover drainage from right to left and vice versa at the level of the ILN, which has been nicely demonstrated in prior lymphoscintigraphy studies [15, 16].

The presence of pelvic lymph node (PLN) metastases is an ominous finding, with a reported 5-year survival rate of 0–66% reported in prior series and 17–54% in those with microscopic lymph node metastasis alone [15, 17–21]. Among patients with ILN metastases, 22–65% will have PLN metastases [22] which can be further stratified among those with 2–3 positive ILN, the probability of PLN metastasis is 23%, and in those with 3 or more positive ILN, the probability rises up to 56% [23]. The PLNs of interest are found along the external iliac vessels and obturator fossa. Up to 12–20 lymph nodes can be found in this area. Unlike crossover which can be seen at the inguinal lymphatic level, crossover from one PLN side to the other contralateral side has not been observed [15]. From a surgical standpoint, the pelvic nodes can be approached in an extraperitoneal fashion using a low midline incision but meticulous control of lymphatic channels with surgical clips and ligation is recommended to minimize the risk of a postoperative pelvic lymphocele. The boundaries of the pelvic lymphadenectomy include the iliac bifurcation proximally, ilioinguinal nerve laterally, and the obturator nerve medially [4, 10]. Patients at risk of harboring PLN metastasis as highlighted in a retrospective study from the Netherlands Cancer

Institute (NCI) included those with 2 or more positive ILN on frozen section, extracapsular nodal extension, and/or poorly differentiated ILN metastases [24].

Pre-surgical Considerations

The importance of identifying lymph node involvement is strongly exhibited in the fact that the 5-year cancer-specific survival is 90–100% in node-negative patients (pN0) after an ILND, and progressively worse in pathologically node-positive patients (16–45%) [25, 26]. Therefore, careful patient selection and stratification are essential, which lead us to the concept of risk-adapted treatment recommendations (i.e., adjuvant systemic chemotherapy +/− radiotherapy, postoperative surveillance strategies). The clinical parameters that help better prognosticate patients include the histopathologic features of the primary tumor including cellular subtype, pathologic stage, and depth of penetration. We know for example that the likelihood of ILN metastatic progression for verrucous carcinoma is 0% vs. 30% for penile SCC (overall) and virtually 100% for basaloid carcinoma [26].

Based on the initial assessment, the treating physician must determine if palpable inguinal adenopathy is in fact present (27) and if so, the specific anatomic location, number of inguinal masses, unilateral or bilateral involvement, dimensions, and mobility or fixation of the ILN to surrounding structures such as the skin, Cooper's ligaments, and/or spermatic cord [4, 11]. Part of the dilemma in the management of penile cancer hinders around the management of palpable inguinal nodes. Previously, the therapeutic dogma was that patients with enlarged inguinal nodes were treated with 4–6 weeks of oral antibiotics as 30–50% of the palpable inguinal lymphadenopathy was secondary to infectious and/or inflammatory reaction and not in fact as a result of ILN metastases. However to avoid a delay in diagnosis, it is now presently recommended to do a fine needle aspiration with ultrasound to establish the diagnosis of ILN metastasis [11, 15]. The clinical premise on which this is based results from our interest to identify those exhibiting a highly aggressive tumor phenotype early on [15, 27]. If the patient is noted or is suspected to have underlying cellulitis at the site of palpable inguinal lymphadenopathy, representing the future site of ILND, then a course of oral antibiotics (potentially intravenous antibiotics based on the antimicrobial sensitivities of the underlying microorganisms) may be helpful [10, 11, 15]. A fine needle aspiration with ultrasound can increase the diagnostic yield in detecting metastatic foci >2 mm in diameter [28–30]. The results of the fine needle aspiration may be negative; therefore based on the clinical suspicion of nodal involvement, an excisional biopsy may be warranted.

The tumor, nodes, and metastasis (TNM) staging for penile cancer was most recently updated by the American Joint Committee on Cancer (AJCC) (Tables 6.1 and 6.2) [31–36]. The revisions have incorporated recommendations and changes from prominent experts worldwide [33, 34, 36]. The AJCC has made the distinction between clinical and pathologic staging and does not take into consideration superficial or deep metastatic lymph nodes, as this may not be differentiated on clinical exam [33]. The most recent TNM staging update incorporated the following changes: the T1 staging category was subdivided into T1a and T1b based on the absence or the presence of lymphovascular invasion or poorly differentiated cancers, T2 constitutes invasion of the corpora cavernosa or spongiosum, T3 now being limited to urethral invasion, and T4 constitutes prostatic invasion [33]. To further characterize penile cancer, it can be defined by the tumor grade (G) which is based on the degree of cellular anaplasia, although there are discrepancies in this regard within the scientific literature. According to the AJCC, grade is defined as follows: GX grade cannot be assessed, G1 well differentiated with no evidence of anaplasia, G2 moderately differentiated (<50% anaplasia), G3 poorly differentiated (>50% anaplastic cells), and G4 undifferentiated [1, 33, 37]. It has been well described that patients with pathologic stage T2 or greater, exhibiting either greater than 50% poorly differentiated cancer or vascular invasion,

Table 6.1 The 2010 tumor, node, metastasis (TNM) of penile cancer [33]

Primary tumor (T)	
TX	Primary tumor cannot be assessed
T0	No evidence of primary tumor
Tis	Carcinoma in situ
Ta	Noninvasive verrucous carcinoma[a]
T1a	Tumor invades subepithelial connective tissue without lymph vascular invasion and is not poorly differentiated (i.e., grade 3–4)
T1b	Tumor invades subepithelial connective tissue with lymph vascular invasion or is poorly differentiated
T2	Tumor invades corpus spongiosum or cavernosum
T3	Tumor invades urethra
T4	Tumor invades other adjacent structures
Regional lymph nodes (N)	
Clinical stage definition[b]	
cNX	Regional lymph nodes cannot be assessed
cN0	No palpable or visibly enlarged inguinal lymph nodes
cN1	Palpable mobile unilateral inguinal lymph nodes
cN2	Palpable mobile multiple or bilateral inguinal lymph nodes
cN3	Palpable fixed inguinal nodal mass or pelvic lymphadenopathy unilateral or bilateral
Pathologic stage definition[c]	
pNX	Regional lymph nodes cannot be assessed
pN0	No regional lymph node metastasis
pN1	Metastasis in a single inguinal lymph node
pN2	Metastasis in multiple or bilateral inguinal lymph nodes
pN3	Extranodal extension of lymph node metastasis or pelvic lymph node(s) unilateral or bilateral
Distant metastasis (M)	
M0	No distant metastasis
M1	Distant metastasis[d]

Used with the permission of the American Joint Committee on Cancer (AJCC), Chicago, IL. The original source for this material is the AJCC Cancer Staging Manual, Seventh Edition (2010), published by Springer Science and Business Media LLC, www.springer.com
[a]Broad pushing penetration (invasion) is permitted; destructive invasion is against diagnosis
[b]Clinical stage definition based on palpation, imaging
[c]Pathologic stage definition based on biopsy or surgical excision
[d]Lymph node metastasis outside of the true pelvis in addition to visceral or bone sites

have a 42–80% risk of nodal metastases, whereby such patients are usually recommended an ILND [1, 15, 38].

Table 6.2 AJCC anatomic stage/prognostic groups [33]

Stage 0	Tis	N0	M0
	Ta	N0	M0
Stage I	T1a	N0	M0
Stage II	T1b	N0	M0
	T2	N0	M0
	T3	N0	M0
Stage IIIa	T1-3	N1	M0
Stage IIIb	T1-3	N2	M0
Stage IV	T4	Any N	M0
	Any T	N3	M0
	Any T	Any N	M1

Used with the permission of the American Joint Committee on Cancer (AJCC), Chicago, Illinois. The original source for this material is the AJCC Cancer Staging Manual, Seventh Edition (2010), published by Springer Science and Business Media LLC, www.springer.com

Table 6.3 EUA guidelines on risk-stratification for nodal metastases in patients with non-palpable ILN [4]

Risk	Stage and grade of primary lesion	Treatment
Low	pTis, pTaG1-2, pT1G1	Surveillance
Intermediate	T1G2	Dependant on vascular growth pattern
High	Any T2 or G3	Lymphadenectomy

It is important to note that in the subset of penile cancer patients not exhibiting palpable inguinal lymphadenopathy, as many as 30% will harbor occult micrometastatic disease to the ILN. To help risk stratify patients and therefore better manage such patients, the European Urological Association (EUA) has defined risk stratification groups based on the primary tumor pathologic stage and grade, with patients stratified into low risk (pTis, pTaG1-2, or pT1G1), intermediate risk (T1G2), and high risk (T2 or G3) as shown in Table 6.3 [4, 39]. For those patients in the intermediate and high-risk categories, the EUA recommend proceeding with an ILND, as the relative risk of harboring inguinal metastasis for low-risk disease is only 4%, whereas it is 34.8% and 45.8% for intermediate- and high-risk groups, respectively [4].

In 2006, Ficarra et al. developed the first nomogram to predict the likelihood of ILN metastasis using primarily the tumor characteristics of the primary penile lesion (tumor thickness, microscopic growth pattern, histological grade,

presence of lymphovascular invasion, tumor infiltration into the corpora cavernosa, corpus spongiosum, or the urethra), and as well the clinic stage of ILN [40]. In the same year, additional nomograms were published to predict the 5-year cancer-specific survival of penile cancer patients [41]. External validation of these statistical models is ongoing, along with the evaluation of potential molecular markers such as p53, E-cadherin, and metalloproteinases (MMP-2 and -9) [42].

In an attempt to enhance clinical staging, a host of imaging modalities have been evaluated and shown to be effective in the diagnostic evaluation of penile cancer patients such as computed tomography (CT) scan and magnetic resonance imaging (MRI). In addition, studies have evaluated the utility of nanoparticle-enhanced MRI, positron emission tomography–CT (PET/CT), and 18F-fluorodeoxyglucose (FDG) PET/CT, yet these prior studies all suffer from their small sample size requiring larger prospective trials to unravel their true benefit [43–47]. Although the diagnostic role of CT and MRI are for the most part limited to patients with non-palpable ILN who may harbor micrometastatic disease, these imaging modalities may decipher if there is any adjacent organ involvement or distant metastasis [29]. The general consensus is that at the present time, MRI with intravenous contrast remains the best diagnostic modality to either corroborate or better characterize the clinical assessment of the inguinal region particularly in patients in whom the physical examination is inaccurate such as in the clinical context of prior surgical resection/scarring, radiotherapy, and/or obesity [45, 48]. The use of 18FDG PET/CT has recently shown great promise as it can provide not only an anatomic but also potential hypermetabolic lesion(s) constituting a suspicious site for occult metastasis. Souillac et al. have recently reported data pertaining to the use of 18FDG PET/CT as a staging tool for invasive penile cancer, especially in patients with clinically impalpable ILN. They as well recommend PET/CT in patients with palpable ILN to enhance the accuracy of clinical staging. By evaluating the presence and extent of metastases, including the involvement of pelvic nodes, this diagnostic modality may drastically optimize our therapeutic approach to penile cancer patients including the potential use of a multimodal approach in patients with bulky or extensive metastatic disease [49]. PET/CT may also be used in the follow-up of patients who initially presented with bulky metastases and underwent upfront salvage chemotherapy in order to assess their treatment response following systemic therapy and help better delineate the curative potential of subsequent ILND; however at this point in time, the clear role of PET/CT in penile cancer remains to be clearly defined [50]. In addition, fine needle aspiration or biopsy can as well serve as an alternate useful diagnostic modality particularly when faced with unclear diagnostic radiographic imaging.

Surgical Treatment

The seminal work of Cabanas in the late 1970s employed lymphatic mapping studies and anatomical dissections to identify the sentinel lymph node among penile cancer patients with non-palpable ILN. Through his work, the lymph node closest to the superficial epigastric vein was determined to be the frequent sentinel node, and if surgically excised and negative for metastasis, Cabanas recommended surgeons not to proceed with an INLD [51]. However, this technique fell out of favor and is no longer recommended, because subsequent studies have not corroborated these early findings with a false-negative rate as high as 25% (9–50%) [4, 52, 53].

The group of Horenblas at the NCI has made a significant contribution in refining the technique and optimizing the performance of dynamic sentinel lymph node biopsy [54]. The technique uses lymphoscintigraphy with technetium^{99m}-labeled nanocolloid, which is injected the day before the procedure at the level of the dermis where the penile lesion is situated or around the penile resection surgical scar. The following day (i.e., day before surgery), a patent blue dye (isosulfan blue) is injected in a similar fashion. The colloid and dye assist in identifying the lymphatic channels, providing a more robust means to identify the sentinel lymph node utilizing two agents to better define the lymphatic pattern of drainage by using the blue dye to determine the suspected

sentinel lymph node upon which a gamma-ray detection probe is applied intra-operatively to determine if this is in fact the lymph node where radiotracer is concentrated supporting this constitutes the sentinel node [55]. Studies by Spiess et al. and others have suggested that the false-negative rate may unfortunately be too high (16–43%) for this technique to be widely recommended. With recent refinements of this technique by the NCI, a false-negative rate as low as 4.9% however can be obtained [54, 56–59]. The technical caveats employed by the NCI group include serial sectioning and immunohistochemical staining of pathological specimens, preoperative ultrasonography with and without fine needle aspiration cytology, and the introduction of exploration of groins in which no sentinel node is visualized on intra-operative assessment [60–62]. The variability in terms of the reported false-negative rates is most likely explained by the learning curve associated with this technique and since there are a limited number of penile cancer cases treated at any single center, it is therefore recommended to perform sentinel lymph node biopsies at tertiary care referral centers which consistently perform at least 20 of these procedures per year [54, 59, 63].

One of the major contributions in decreasing the morbidity associated with ILND is credited to Catalona in 1988, in which he defined the modified ILND template. By using shorter skin incisions, limiting the area of dissection not including the area lateral to the femoral artery and caudal to the fossa ovalis, and preserving the saphenous vein with no muscle flap transposition, this technique decreased the morbidity while maintaining the desired oncological outcomes. The suitable patient for this approach is a patient that has clinically negative ILN in the context of an increased risk for ILN metastasis based on his primary penile tumor pathologic characteristics. The skin incision and subcutaneous tissue dissection should be conducted preserving the superficial blood supply to the skin flaps, thus avoiding the risk of postoperative skin necrosis, infection, and wound breakdown. After the skin incision is made, a surgical plane is developed beneath Scarpa's fascia. The superior boundary of the ILND is established at this point and

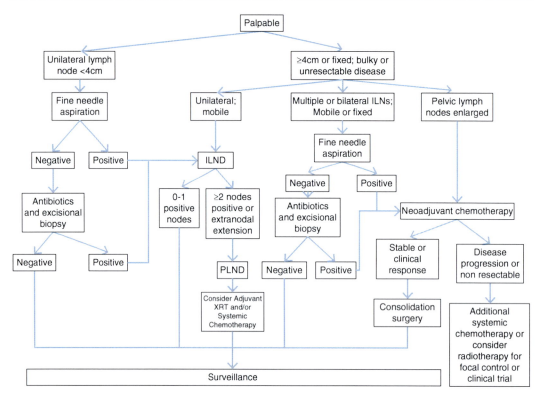

Fig. 6.1 Management algorithm of ILN in patients with penile SCC

extends to the level of the external oblique fascia, the external inguinal ring, and spermatic cord. The first lymphatic packet is obtained with meticulous control of lymphatics, and extends from the base of the penis to the superomedial portion of this lymph node package. The superficial and deep inguinal nodes are then resected using the adductor longus muscle at the medial boundary of dissection and the femoral artery as the lateral boundary. The saphenous vein is identified and preserved using a modified ILND template minimizing the likelihood and extent of postoperative lymphedema. Further dissection is carried caudally to the level of the skin flap dissection and the final packet is sent for frozen section and final pathologic evaluation assessing if any positive lymph node(s) is present and the total number of lymph nodes resected. At the end of the surgical dissection, a closed-suction drain is placed, and the incision is closed in a standard multilayer fashion [10, 64]. By targeting the superomedial quadrant of the inguinal region, it is felt that this

approach can maintain excellent oncological outcomes as this is the most frequent site of ILN metastasis while decreasing the morbidity of the procedure by limiting the length of the incision, amount of surgical dissection, and amount of loco-regional lymphatic drainage of the lower extremities disturbed [14, 65]. An important caveat is that we recommend each lymph node package be sent for frozen section as the surgical procedure should be converted to a full standard ILND if any positive lymph nodes are found on frozen section.

Patients who present with biopsy-proven ILN metastasis (particularly if bulky ≥3 cm or if fixed to the surrounding structures) should be considered for neoadjuvant systemic chemotherapy with a summary of our surgical approach highlighted in Fig. 6.1. Recent studies have highlighted the favorable oncologic outcomes in patients who receive upfront systemic chemotherapy followed by surgical consolidation among patients with bulky inguinal lymph

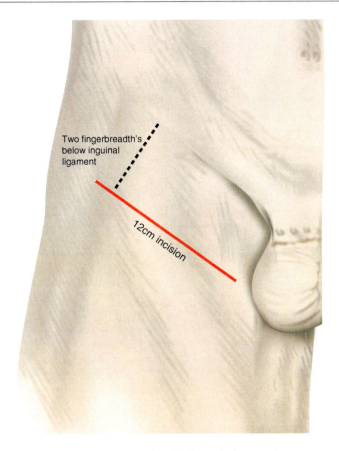

Two fingerbreadth's below inguinal ligament

12cm incision

Fig. 6.2 Schematic diagram highlighting our standardized ILND surgical approach

metastasis [66, 67]. The boundaries of this dissection are defined by a line taken from the external ring to the anterior superior iliac spine (superior boundary), along a vertical line extending from the anterior superior iliac spine downwards 20 cm (inferolateral boundary), and a line drawn from the pubic tubercle 15 cm vertically downwards (medial boundary). Different types of surgical incisions have been described and recommended, including an elliptical incision, S-shaped incision, and an incision parallel to the inguinal ligament but typically 2–3 fingerbreadths below it (Fig. 6.2). Elliptical incisions with resection of overlying skin and superficial layers should be considered when a resection of the overlying skin either directly invaded by the tumor or broken down by infection/tumor/prior therapy is noted. The same surgical principles as

with the modified template are adhered to, ensuring that the skin flaps are well developed with preservation of their blood supply. Several incision techniques have been described, including a Gibson incision, S-shaped, T-shaped, horizontal, and straight. Ornellas et al. based on their series of 200 ILND suggested a benefit of a Gibson incision over an S-shaped incision with a lower risk of wound complications (72% vs. 82%, respectively) [68, 69]. When comparing the T-shaped incision to a horizontal incision, Ravi et al. reported an increase in the incidence of flap necrosis with the T-shape incision [70]. A series from Bouchot et al. also evaluated the horizontal incision and noted a 3–5% decrease in flap necrosis rates [71]. Yao et al. recently assessed a closer look at the anatomy, particularly the vessels that supply the skin of the area, and based on this

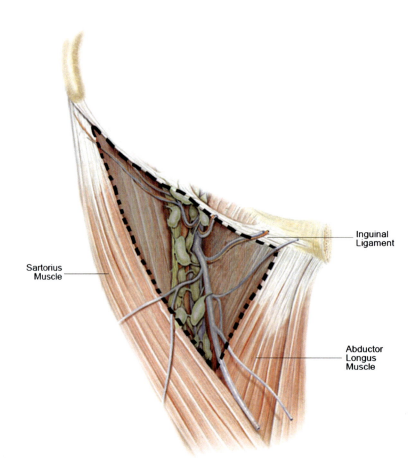

Sartorius
Muscle

Inguinal
Ligament

Abductor
Longus
Muscle

Fig. 6.3 Illustration depicting the anatomical boundaries of dissection for ILND

and other studies used a modified technique with an S-shaped incision, using anatomical landmarks to separate the layers and preserving the fascia lata, reporting a lower complication rate without adversely impacting oncologic effectiveness [72, 73]. The authors describe the incision as an S-shaped that is shorter and more oblique, providing satisfactory exposure without placing excess tension on the skin flaps and preserving the subdermal plexus that directly supplies the skin and adjacent vascular territories of the skin flaps [72]. The incision may also be done in an elliptical fashion over the inguinal nodes as described by Kean et al. who excise a 4-cm-wide skin segment over the ILN specimen [74]. The lymph node dissection is carried down from the superior boundary of the external oblique aponeu-

rosis and the spermatic cord to the inferior border of the inguinal ligament. The long saphenous vein is found within the femoral triangle, where it is identified and ligated. Next, the dissection is carried down through the fascia lata overlying the sartorius muscle laterally and medially through the thinner fascia of the adductor longus muscle (Fig. 6.3). The surgical dissection is continued along the femoral vessels superiorly until the femoral canal is reached, where access to the pelvis can be easily attained enabling a concomitant PLN dissection to be performed if clinically indicated. At the level of the sapheno-femoral junction, the saphenous vein is ligated as part of this approach. A careful and meticulous surgical technique is used to minimize injury to the femoral nerve and profunda femoris artery by not exposing if possible and preserving them within the iliacus fascia. The sartorius muscle can be transposed once the superficial and deep ILND is completed by detaching its attachments from the anterior superior iliac spine, enabling to provide myocutaneous coverage over the femoral vessels termed a sartorius rotation flap [10].

A closed-suction drain is placed prior to the completion of the surgical procedure, and the skin is thereafter closed with the muscle and subcutaneous tissues reapproximated to help obliterate any potential dead space for a postoperative fluid collection to accumulate which may serve as a nidus for infection or lymphocele formation [10, 75]. The closed-suction drain is removed when there is minimal drainage (typically <30–50 mL/day output over consecutive shifts) which typically occurs 3–17 days following surgery [10, 75, 76]. Postoperatively, patients are typically maintained on bed rest for 48–72 h particularly if a myocutaneous and/or large skin flap(s) is employed. The use of oral perioperative antibiotics (cephalosporin or other gram-positive broad-spectrum coverage) has been shown to decrease the risk of wound infections in this patient cohort and can improve wound healing [10].

The conception that minimally invasive surgical techniques including video endoscopy inguinal lymphadenectomy (VEIL) and robotic assisted laparoscopic ILND could be employed in the first-line surgical armamentarium to penile cancer is an active area of research and debate which will be discussed in a subsequent chapter. These surgical approaches offer the potential for fewer cutaneous complications while likely do not compromise oncologic outcomes although rigorous scientific data is currently lacking [77–79]. In 2003, Bishoff et al. described a laparoscopic approach to a modified ILND template in two cadavers and in one patient with clinical stage T3N1M0 penile cancer. The anatomical dissection in the cadavers was limited secondary to the few number of lymph nodes present close to the femoral vessels [80]. When considering a patient for a laparoscopic procedure, the same surgical and oncologic principles should be adhered to as with the open approach. Patients

who may be ideal suitable candidates for such an approach include penile cancer patients with non-palpable ILN and aggressive primary tumor pathological features (≥T2, presence of high-grade cancer and/or vascular invasion). The anatomical boundaries of the minimally invasive ILND follow the modified template as described by Catalona et al. [64], with the difference with the VEIL technique being that the saphenous vein is not always preserved. The limits of the dissection are the traditional anatomic boundaries of the sartorius muscle laterally, the adductor longus muscle medially, and the inguinal ligament and spermatic cord superiorly [81]. Compression stockings are employed at anesthesia induction and continued throughout the perioperative period [81]. Tobias-Machado et al. in their surgical series compared open ILND with a VEIL procedure employing a modified template as described by Bishoff in penile cancer patients with non-palpable inguinal lymphadenopathy [79]. In their series, the authors reported favorable oncologic and cosmetic results, as they were able to dissect and excise the same number of lymph nodes on the laparoscopic side as on the open ILND side in ten patients following a mean of 18.7 months, with no reported recurrences or cases of disease progression [79]. From the patients' perspective, increased pain was reported in the open procedure arm. Tobias-Machado et al. conducted a comparable study in 20 limbs that underwent a VEIL procedure and 10 that underwent an open procedure. The results favored the VEIL procedure arm with complication rates of 20% with the VEIL procedure as compared to 70% with the open procedure [77]. Sotelo and colleagues were as well early proponents of the VEIL procedure. They used this laparoscopic approach in eight patients (14 ILND) and in this series, there were no perioperative or wound-related complications, with the development of lymphoceles in 3 groins (23%) [82]. It is evident that more efforts are desperately needed to validate this minimally invasive technique as its initial short- to intermediate-term results are encouraging in our constant pursuit to optimize surgical outcomes while never compromising oncologic principles.

Recommendations for Minimizing the Risk of Complications

Traditionally, ILND has been plagued by high complication rates (80–100%) [69, 70]. Steps may be taken to minimize the risk of these perioperative complications. Bevan-Thomas et al. [83] reported on a novel categorization of complications specific to penile cancer surgery, with minor complications encompassing a local wound debridement in the clinic, mild (trace +1) pitting edema to moderate (+2) leg edema, seroma formation not requiring aspiration, and minimal skin edge necrosis requiring no surgical intervention. In contrast, major complications were categorized as severe leg edema interfering with ambulation, skin flap necrosis requiring a skin graft, rehospitalization for wound care, wound care or sepsis requiring intravenous antibiotics, deep venous thrombosis (DVT) or pulmonary embolus (PE), surgical re-exploration or invasive procedure (incision and drainage of abscess or seroma), and death [83]. Radical ILND series have reported minor complications in 40–54% of dissections [71, 76, 83, 84] and major complications in 5–21%

[76, 83, 84]. Contemporary series using modified templates of dissection and improved surgical techniques report minor complications including seroma (25–27%), lymphorrhea (9–10%), and wound infection or skin necrosis (0–9%), as shown in Tables 6.4 and 6.5 [70, 71, 76, 83–90].

The surgeon can minimize the risk of complications by being meticulous at each step of the perioperative care as highlighted in a recent review by Spiess et al. [27]. Attempts to minimize the risk of surgical complications begin in the preoperative holding area, with DVT and infection precautions. Both historical and contemporary series report similar incidences of DVT and PE, with a reported incidence ranging between 5 and 7% [70, 76]. To obviate this risk, patients should have compression stockings or sequential pneumatic compression devices placed prior to anesthesia induction. The compression stockings and sequential compression devices should be continued while the patient is maintained on bed rest postoperatively [91, 92]. In the perioperative period, patients with a remote history of a DVT/PE should be started on low-molecular-weight heparin (LMWH) as soon as it is determined that this is safe from a minimal

Table 6.4 Morbidity of radical ILND

Study	No. ILND	% Infection	% Skin necrosis	% Lymphedema	% Seroma	% Lymphocele
Ravi [70]	405	16.3	62	26.7	6.9	9
Ayyappan et al. [87]	135	70	36	57	12	87
Bevan-Thomas et al. [83]	40	15	12.5	25	7.5	5
Bouchot et al. [71]	58	6.9	12	22.4	13.8	5.2
Nelson et al. [84]	80	7.5	10	15	0	15
d'Ancona et al. [89]	8	0	37.5	37.5	37.5	12.5
Spiess et al. [76]	86	9	11	17	0	2
Yao et al. [72]	150	1.4	4.7	13.9	2	2

Table 6.5 Morbidity of modified ILND

Study	No. ILND	% Infection	% Skin necrosis	% Lymphedema	% Seroma	% Lymphocele
Catalona [64]	12	0	8.3	100	0	8.3
Parra [86]	24	0	0	8.3	0	4.2
Cobentz and Theodorescu [90]	22	4.5	4.5	36.4	0	22.7
Bevan-Thomas et al. [83]	66	9.1	4.5	21.2	12.1	0
Bouchot et al. [71]	118	0.8	2.5	3.4	2.5	0
d'Ancona et al. [89]	42	0	0	0	26.3	10.5

postoperative bleeding risk standpoint. When a patient presents with a history of DVT/PE within the last 6 months, it is encouraged to initiate DVT/PE prophylaxis preoperatively in concert with internal medicine or hematology recommendations and thereafter for 28 days from the date of surgery with a low-dose LMWH which is then transitioned to an oral anticoagulation agent in the outpatient setting typically for at least 6 months [76]. In a series from Sawczuk et al. they had a zero complication rate specifically pertaining to DVT/PE or significant bleeding risk when they used LMWH for DVT prophylaxis in patients undergoing urologic oncologic surgical procedures [92]. Based on the extent of the surgical dissection, the duration of postoperative bed rest can be tailored; with procedures where a limited surgical dissection not employing a myocutaneous flap is conducted, earlier ambulation after as little as 8 h of postoperative bed rest can be considered [76, 84].

A dose of preoperative intravenous antibiotics (e.g., ampicillin/gentamycin or ampicillin/ciprofloxacin) should be administered prior to starting the surgical procedure and the antibiotic should encompass at least the most commonly encountered bacteria within inguinal wounds, i.e., gram-negative rods, Staphylococcus species, diphtheroids, and Peptostreptococcus. If there is a concern for a skin infection at the site of the procedure, then a wound culture should be obtained to identify the potentially offending organisms and target antibiotic therapy before any surgical procedure is conducted [76]. When there is skin breakdown prior to surgery, attempts should be made to manage any infection, necrosis, and local wound issues prior to proceeding with ILND. In this regard, the patient should be covered with antibiotic therapy prophylactically prior to surgery and then into the perioperative recovery period until there are no signs of obvious infections and all subcutaneous drains have been removed [11, 76, 93].

Once in the operative room, there are several parameters that the surgeon can enhance to help minimize the risk of complications resulting from ILND. In order to optimize the patient's surgical outcomes, certain appropriate preoperative precautions can be undertaken and surgical techniques/concepts must be adhered to. In a study

assessing the skin preparation of patients undergoing clean-contaminated surgical procedures, Darouiche et al. determined that preoperative skin preparation with a chlorhexidine–alcohol scrub provided a significantly lower surgical site infection rate at 30 days when compared to a skin prep with a povidone–iodine solution (9.5% vs. 16.1%, respectively; $P = 0.004$) [94].

The decision of how the skin and subcutaneous tissues are dissected and manipulated is pivotal. Throughout the procedure, meticulous atraumatic handling of all tissues cannot be overemphasized, as this will help preserve the superficial subcutaneous tissue (fibrous layer) of Camper's fascia. If the skin flap is made too thin, then there is an increased risk of wound-related issues including ischemia, necrosis, and wound dehiscence [11, 76]. During the ILND, control of all visible lymphatic channels can significantly decrease the risk of lymphocele and/or hematoma formation which can be further enhanced by the preservation of the saphenous vein as described by Catalona. In addition, the preservation of the saphenous vein renders this vessel available for potential future venous harvesting and grafting if cardiovascular or peripheral vascular surgical procedures are required [64, 76]. Control of lymphatic channels throughout the ILND can be achieved with small absorbable suture or titanium surgical clips [75, 76]. The use of a LigaSure™ device (Covidien; Boulder, Colorado) may as well seal and cut lymphatic channels with the added benefit to reduce the operative time as described by Gallo Rolania et al. [95]. Another option albeit infrequently utilized is to perform lympho-venous anastomoses immediately after the completion of the ILND as Orifice et al. described reporting a reduction in lymphedema and length of hospital stay [96].

Awareness of the local vasculature anatomy (arterial and venous) is essential to reduce the risk of postoperative major vascular injury, bleeding, and hematoma formation. Contemporary series have reported a 2–4% risk of vascular injury or hematoma at the time of ILND [76, 83]. Any active bleeding in the postoperative setting warrants immediate surgical exploration to evacuate the clot and find the source of bleeding in order to minimize the risk of infection and promote wound healing particularly if the patient demonstrates any hemodynamic instability or concern of a wound infection [76].

Depending on the skin and subcutaneous defect resulting from the ILND, the skin may be approximated primarily if a very small defect (<1–2 cm in largest diameter) results typically when only a superficial ILND is conducted on this ipsilateral side; yet if the defect is too large or if there is concern of direct exposure of the femoral vessels, a rotational scrotal skin flap or an abdominal wall advancement flap may be necessary [70]. With more extensive defects (typically resulting from a concomitant superficial and deep ILND), a myocutaneous flap usually a sartorius muscle rotational flap, internal oblique, rectus abdominis, pedicled anterolateral thigh [97], and gracilis tensor fascia lata flaps may be required [76, 98].

Post-op Care: Surveillance Strategies, Management of Local, Regional, Metastatic Recurrences

The goal of surgical management of inguinal or PLN metastasis is twofold serving both a diagnostic and therapeutic role. Postoperative surveillance care of such patients is essential to ensure that there is no disease recurrence and if so, they are recognized early at a time they are potentially curable, as well as to ensure that the patient is healing adequately. A good follow-up regimen assists with the early detection of any recurrence, thus avoiding a delay in diagnosis. Most recurrences will occur within the first two years. Since penile cancer will metastasize in a predictable fashion, those patients with clinically negative inguinal nodes (Nx) should be monitored every 6 months for years 1 and 2, and then every 12 months for years 3–5 with a thorough examination of the penis and bilateral inguinal regions. If there are concerns with the ability to perform a good physical exam (obese patients or those who have previously undergone inguinal dissections), imaging with ultrasound, CT, or MRI should be considered. Patients with no metastasis or metastasis to a single node (N0 or N1) are to be monitored every 6 months during the first 2 years, and then on an annual basis through year 5. Positive lymph node involvement of multiple sites and extension of nodal involvement (N2 and N3) require more stringent surveillance with clinical examination and imaging. A clinical assessment should be done every 3 months for the first 2 years, and then every 6–12 months through year 5. Imaging recommendations for these patients should include a chest CT or X-ray every 3–6 months during the first 2 years, along with an abdominal and pelvic CT or MRI every 3–6 months for the first 2 years, and then every 6–12 months through year 5.

A delay in diagnosis adversely impacts survival, with a median survival of less than 6 months among those with a recurrence in the inguinal region; therefore close follow-up will help in the early detection of such recurrences. Careful review of the patient's postoperative course, quality of life, and extent of disease recurrence will delineate if the patient is a good candidate for salvage treatments with systemic chemotherapy, external beam radiation therapy, salvage surgery, or a combination of these modalities [11, 99].

Conclusion

The surgical management of inguinal lymph node metastases secondary to penile cancer has been fraught with much fear due to its traditionally high perioperative morbidity. Yet, it has been well described that early detection and surgical management of inguinal metastasis among penile cancer patients can be curative. Therefore, we must continue to build on the progress made by our peers in maintaining excellent oncologic outcomes while continually reducing the perioperative risk of complications. Lastly, minimally invasive surgical approaches to penile cancer may continue to redefine our therapeutic approach to ILN in the clinical context of penile cancer provided we continually adhere to our fundamental surgical oncologic principles.

References

1. Slaton JW, Morgenstern N, Levy DA, Santos Jr MW, Tamboli P, Ro JY, et al. Tumor stage, vascular invasion and the percentage of poorly differentiated cancer: independent prognosticators for inguinal lymph node metastasis in penile squamous cancer. J Urol. 2001;165(4):1138–42.

2. Daling JR, Madeleine MM, Johnson LG, Schwartz SM, Shera KA, Wurscher MA, et al. Penile cancer: importance of circumcision, human papillomavirus and smoking in in situ and invasive disease. Int J Cancer. 2005;116(4):606–16.

3. Horenblas S, van Tinteren H, Delemarre JF, Moonen LM, Lustig V, van Waardenburg EW. Squamous cell carcinoma of the penis. III. Treatment of regional lymph nodes. J Urol. 1993;149(3):492–7.

4. Pizzocaro G, Algaba F, Horenblas S, Solsona E, Tana S, Van Der Poel H, et al. EAU penile cancer guidelines 2009. Eur Urol. 2010;57(6):1002–12.

5. Stancik I, Holtl W. Penile cancer: review of the recent literature. Curr Opin Urol. 2003;13(6):467–72.

6. Kroon BK, Horenblas S, Lont AP, Tanis PJ, Gallee MP, Nieweg OE. Patients with penile carcinoma benefit from immediate resection of clinically occult lymph node metastases. J Urol. 2005;173(3):816–9.

7. Svatek RS, Munsell M, Kincaid JM, Hegarty P, Slaton JW, Busby JE, et al. Association between lymph node density and disease specific survival in patients with penile cancer. J Urol. 2009;182(6):2721–7.

8. Pettaway C, Lynch Jr D, Davis J. Tumors of the penis. In: Wein AJ, Kavoussi L, Novick AC, Partin AW, Peters CA, editors. Campbell-Walsh urology. 9th ed. Philadelphia: Saunders; 2007. p. 959–92.

9. Daseler EH, Anson BJ, Reimann AF. Radical excision of the inguinal and iliac lymph glands; a study based upon 450 anatomical dissections and upon supportive clinical observations. Surg Gynecol Obstet. 1948;87(6):679–94.

10. Sharp DS, Angermeier KW. Surgery of penile and urethral carcinoma. In: Wein AJ, Kavoussi L, Novick AC, Partin AW, Peters CA, editors. Campbell-Walsh urology. 9th ed. Philadelphia: Saunders; 2007. p. 993–1022.

11. Heyns CF, Fleshner N, Sangar V, Schlenker B, Yuvaraja TB, van Poppel H. Management of the lymph nodes in penile cancer. Urology. 2010;76(2 Suppl 1):S43–57.

12. Loughlin KR. Surgical atlas. Surgical management of penile carcinoma: the inguinal nodes. BJU Int. 2006;97(5):1125–34.

13. Wood HM, Angermeier KW. Anatomic considerations of the penis, lymphatic drainage, and biopsy of the sentinel node. Urol Clin North Am. 2010;37(3):327–34.

14. Protzel C, Alcaraz A, Horenblas S, Pizzocaro G, Zlotta A, Hakenberg OW. Lymphadenectomy in the surgical management of penile cancer. Eur Urol. 2009;55(5):1075–88.

15. Horenblas S. Lymphadenectomy for squamous cell carcinoma of the penis. Part 1: diagnosis of lymph node metastasis. BJU Int. 2001;88(5):467–72.

16. Kroon BK, Valdes Olmos RA, van Tinteren H, Nieweg OE, Horenblas S. Reproducibility of lymphoscintigraphy for lymphatic mapping in patients with penile carcinoma. J Urol. 2005;174(6):2214–7.

17. Srinivas V, Morse MJ, Herr HW, Sogani PC, Whitmore Jr WF. Penile cancer: relation of extent of nodal metastasis to survival. J Urol. 1987;137(5):880–2.

18. Pow-Sang JE, Benavente V, Pow-Sang JM, Pow-Sang M. Bilateral ilioinguinal lymph node dissection in the management of cancer of the penis. Semin Surg Oncol. 1990;6(4):241–2.

19. Ravi R. Correlation between the extent of nodal involvement and survival following groin dissection for carcinoma of the penis. Br J Urol. 1993;72(5 Pt 2):817–9.

20. Sanchez-Ortiz RF, Pettaway CA. The role of lymphadenectomy in penile cancer. Urol Oncol. 2004;22(3):236–44. discussion 44–5.

21. Lopes A, Bezerra AL, Serrano SV, Hidalgo GS. Iliac nodal metastases from carcinoma of the penis treated surgically. BJU Int. 2000;86(6):690–3.

22. Leijte JA, Kirrander P, Antonini N, Windahl T, Horenblas S. Recurrence patterns of squamous cell carcinoma of the penis: recommendations for follow-up based on a two-centre analysis of 700 patients. Eur Urol. 2008;54(1):161–8.

23. Culkin DJ, Beer TM. Advanced penile carcinoma. J Urol. 2003;170(2 Pt 1):359–65.

24. Lont AP, Kroon BK, Gallee MP, van Tinteren H, Moonen LM, Horenblas S. Pelvic lymph node dissection for penile carcinoma: extent of inguinal lymph node involvement as an indicator for pelvic lymph node involvement and survival. J Urol. 2007;177(3):947–52. discussion 52.

25. Campbell MF, Wein AJ, Kavoussi LR. Campbell-Walsh urology. In: Alan J. Wein, Louis R. Kavoussi, editors. 9th ed. Philadelphia: Saunders; 2007. p. 4 v. (xlii, 3945, cxv p.).

26. Ficarra V, Akduman B, Bouchot O, Palou J, Tobias-Machado M. Prognostic factors in penile cancer. Urology. 2010;76(2 Suppl 1):S66–73.

27. Margulis V, Sagalowsky AI. Penile cancer: management of regional lymphatic drainage. Urol Clin North Am. 2010;37(3):411–9.

28. Hadway P, Smith Y, Corbishley C, Heenan S, Watkin NA. Evaluation of dynamic lymphoscintigraphy and sentinel lymph-node biopsy for detecting occult metastases in patients with penile squamous cell carcinoma. BJU Int. 2007;100(3):561–5.

29. Hughes B, Leijte J, Shabbir M, Watkin N, Horenblas S. Non-invasive and minimally invasive staging of regional lymph nodes in penile cancer. World J Urol. 2009;27(2):197–203.

30. Kroon BK, Horenblas S, Deurloo EE, Nieweg OE, Teertstra HJ. Ultrasonography-guided fine-needle aspiration cytology before sentinel node biopsy in patients with penile carcinoma. BJU Int. 2005;95(4):517–21.

31. Leijte JA, Horenblas S. Shortcomings of the current TNM classification for penile carcinoma: time for a change? World J Urol. 2009;27(2):151–4.

32. The National Cancer Institute, Penile Cancer Treatment. [cited 2012]; Available from: http://www.cancer.gov/cancertopics/types/penile.

33. Edge SB, Byrd DR, Compton CC, More A, More A, More A, et al. Penis. In: Edge SB, Byrd DR, Compton CC, More A, More A, More A, et al., editors. AJCC cancer staging manual. 7th ed. New York, NY: Springer; 2010. p. 449–50.

34. Barocas DA, Chang SS. Penile cancer: clinical presentation, diagnosis, and staging. Urol Clin North Am. 2010;37(3):343–52.

35. Sobin LH, Wittekind C. International Union against cancer. TNM classification of malignant tumours. 6th ed. New York: Wiley-Liss; 2002.

36. Leijte JA, Gallee M, Antonini N, Horenblas S. Evaluation of current TNM classification of penile carcinoma. J Urol. 2008;180(3):933–8. discussion 8.

37. Velazquez EF, Ayala G, Liu H, Chaux A, Zanotti M, Torres J, et al. Histologic grade and perineural invasion are more important than tumor thickness as predictor of nodal metastasis in penile squamous cell carcinoma invading 5 to 10 mm. Am J Surg Pathol. 2008;32(7):974–9.

38. Bhagat SK, Gopalakrishnan G, Kekre NS, Chacko NK, Kumar S, Manipadam MT, et al. Factors predicting inguinal node metastasis in squamous cell cancer of penis. World J Urol. 2010;28(1):93–8.

39. Solsona E, Iborra I, Rubio J, Casanova JL, Ricos JV, Calabuig C. Prospective validation of the association of local tumor stage and grade as a predictive factor for occult lymph node micrometastasis in patients with penile carcinoma and clinically negative inguinal lymph nodes. J Urol. 2001;165(5):1506–9.

40. Ficarra V, Zattoni F, Artibani W, Fandella A, Martignoni G, Novara G, et al. Nomogram predictive of pathological inguinal lymph node involvement in patients with squamous cell carcinoma of the penis. J Urol. 2006;175(5):1700–4. discussion 4–5.

41. Kattan MW, Ficarra V, Artibani W, Cunico SC, Fandella A, Martignoni G, et al. Nomogram predictive of cancer specific survival in patients undergoing partial or total amputation for squamous cell carcinoma of the penis. J Urol. 2006;175(6):2103–8. discussion 8.

42. Novara G, Galfano A, De Marco V, Artibani W, Ficarra V. Prognostic factors in squamous cell carcinoma of the penis. Nat Clin Pract Urol. 2007;4(3):140–6.

43. Scher B, Seitz M, Albinger W, Reiser M, Schlenker B, Stief C, et al. Value of PET and PET/CT in the diagnostics of prostate and penile cancer. Recent Results Cancer Res. 2008;170:159–79.

44. Schlenker B, Scher B, Tiling R, Siegert S, Hungerhuber E, Gratzke C, et al. Detection of inguinal lymph node involvement in penile squamous cell carcinoma by 18F-fluorodeoxyglucose PET/CT: A prospective single-center study. Urol Oncol. 2012; Jan–Feb; 30(1):55–9.

45. Mueller-Lisse UG, Scher B, Scherr MK, Seitz M. Functional imaging in penile cancer: PET/computed tomography, MRI, and sentinel lymph node biopsy. Curr Opin Urol. 2008;18(1):105–10.

46. Scher B, Seitz M, Reiser M, Hungerhuber E, Hahn K, Tiling R, et al. 18F-FDG PET/CT for staging of penile cancer. J Nucl Med. 2005;46(9):1460–5.

47. Tabatabaei S, Harisinghani M, McDougal WS. Regional lymph node staging using lymphotropic nanoparticle enhanced magnetic resonance imaging with ferumoxtran-10 in patients with penile cancer. J Urol. 2005;174(3):923–7. discussion 7.

48. Caso JR, Rodriguez AR, Correa J, Spiess PE. Update in the management of penile cancer. Int Braz J Urol. 2009;35(4):406–15.

49. Souillac I, Rigaud J, Ansquer C, Marconnet L, Bouchot O. Prospective evaluation of (18) F-fluorodeoxyglucose positron emission tomography-computerized tomography to assess inguinal lymph node status in invasive squamous cell carcinoma of the penis. J Urol. 2012;187(2):493–7.

50. Graafland NM, Valdes Olmos RA, Teertstra HJ, Kerst JM, Bergman AM, Horenblas S. 18F-FDG PET/CT for monitoring induction chemotherapy in patients with primary inoperable penile carcinoma: first clinical results. Eur J Nucl Med Mol Imaging. 2010; 37(8):1474–80.

51. Cabanas RM. An approach for the treatment of penile carcinoma. Cancer. 1977;39(2):456–66.

52. Pettaway CA, Pisters LL, Dinney CP, Jularbal F, Swanson DA, von Eschenbach AC, et al. Sentinel lymph node dissection for penile carcinoma: the M.D. Anderson Cancer Center experience. J Urol. 1995; 154(6):1999–2003.

53. Wespes E, Simon J, Schulman CC. Cabanas approach: is sentinel node biopsy reliable for staging penile carcinoma? Urology. 1986;28(4):278–9.

54. Leijte JA, Kroon BK, Valdes Olmos RA, Nieweg OE, Horenblas S. Reliability and safety of current dynamic sentinel node biopsy for penile carcinoma. Eur Urol. 2007;52(1):170–7.

55. Valdes Olmos RA, Tanis PJ, Hoefnagel CA, Jansen L, Nieweg OE, Meinhardt W, et al. Penile lymphoscintigraphy for sentinel node identification. Eur J Nucl Med. 2001;28(5):581–5.

56. Kroon BK, Horenblas S, Meinhardt W, van der Poel HG, Bex A, van Tinteren H, et al. Dynamic sentinel node biopsy in penile carcinoma: evaluation of 10 years experience. Eur Urol. 2005;47(5):601–6. discussion 6.

57. Tanis PJ, Lont AP, Meinhardt W, Olmos RA, Nieweg OE, Horenblas S. Dynamic sentinel node biopsy for penile cancer: reliability of a staging technique. J Urol. 2002;168(1):76–80.

58. Gonzaga-Silva LF, Tavares JM, Freitas FC, Tomas Filho ME, Oliveira VP, Lima MV. The isolated gamma probe technique for sentinel node penile carcinoma detection is unreliable. Int Braz J Urol. 2007;33(1):58–63. discussion 4–7.

59. Spiess PE, Izawa JI, Bassett R, Kedar D, Busby JE, Wong F, et al. Preoperative lymphoscintigraphy and dynamic sentinel node biopsy for staging penile cancer: results with pathological correlation. J Urol. 2007;177(6):2157–61.

60. Kroon BK, Horenblas S, Estourgie SH, Lont AP, Valdes Olmos RA, Nieweg OE. How to avoid false-negative dynamic sentinel node procedures in penile carcinoma. J Urol. 2004;171(6 Pt 1):2191–4.

61. Lont AP, Horenblas S, Tanis PJ, Gallee MP, van Tinteren H, Nieweg OE. Management of clinically node negative penile carcinoma: improved survival after the introduction of dynamic sentinel node biopsy. J Urol. 2003;170(3):783–6.

62. Kroon BK, Lont AP, Valdes Olmos RA, Nieweg OE, Horenblas S. Morbidity of dynamic sentinel node biopsy in penile carcinoma. J Urol. 2005;173(3):813–5.

63. Ficarra V, Galfano A. Should the dynamic sentinel node biopsy (DSNB) be considered the gold standard in the evaluation of lymph node status in patients with penile carcinoma? Eur Urol. 2007;52(1):17–9. discussion 20-1.

64. Catalona WJ. Modified inguinal lymphadenectomy for carcinoma of the penis with preservation of saphenous veins: technique and preliminary results. J Urol. 1988;140(2):306–10.

65. Lopes A, Rossi BM, Fonseca FP, Morini S. Unreliability of modified inguinal lymphadenectomy for clinical staging of penile carcinoma. Cancer. 1996;77(10):2099–102.

66. Bermejo C, Busby JE, Spiess PE, Heller L, Pagliaro LC, Pettaway CA. Neoadjuvant chemotherapy followed by aggressive surgical consolidation for metastatic penile squamous cell carcinoma. J Urol. 2007; 177(4):1335–8.

67. Pagliaro LC, Crook J. Multimodality therapy in penile cancer: when and which treatments? World J Urol. 2009;27(2):221–5.

68. Ornellas AA. Management of penile cancer. J Surg Oncol. 2008;97(3):199–200.

69. Ornellas AA, Seixas AL, de Moraes JR. Analyses of 200 lymphadenectomies in patients with penile carcinoma. J Urol. 1991;146(2):330–2.

70. Ravi R. Morbidity following groin dissection for penile carcinoma. Br J Urol. 1993;72(6):941–5.

71. Bouchot O, Rigaud J, Maillet F, Hetet JF, Karam G. Morbidity of inguinal lymphadenectomy for invasive penile carcinoma. Eur Urol. 2004;45(6):761–5. discussion 5–6.

72. Yao K, Tu H, Li YH, Qin ZK, Liu ZW, Zhou FJ, et al. Modified technique of radical inguinal lymphadenectomy for penile carcinoma: morbidity and outcome. J Urol. 2010;184(2):546–52.

73. Zhang Q, Qiao Q, Gould LJ, Myers WT, Phillips LG. Study of the neural and vascular anatomy of the anterolateral thigh flap. J Plast Reconstr Aesthet Surg. 2010;63(2):365–71.

74. Kean J, Hough M, Stevenson JH. Skin excision and groin lymphadenectomy: techniques and outcomes. Lymphology. 2006;39(3):141–6.

75. Crawford ED, Daneshgari F. Management of regional lymphatic drainage in carcinoma of the penis. Urol Clin North Am. 1992;19(2):305–17.

76. Spiess PE, Hernandez MS, Pettaway CA. Contemporary inguinal lymph node dissection: minimizing complications. World J Urol. 2009;27(2):205–12.

77. Tobias-Machado M, Tavares A, Silva MN, Molina Jr WR, Forseto PH, Juliano RV, et al. Can video endoscopic inguinal lymphadenectomy achieve a lower morbidity than open lymph node dissection in penile cancer patients? J Endourol. 2008;22(8):1687–91.

78. Tobias-Machado M, Tavares A, Ornellas AA, Molina Jr WR, Juliano RV, Wroclawski ER. Video endoscopic inguinal lymphadenectomy: a new minimally invasive procedure for radical management of inguinal nodes in patients with penile squamous cell carcinoma. J Urol. 2007;177(3):953–7. discussion 8.

79. Tobias-Machado M, Tavares A, Molina Jr WR, Forseto Jr PH, Juliano RV, Wroclawski ER. Video endoscopic inguinal lymphadenectomy (VEIL): minimally invasive resection of inguinal lymph nodes. Int Braz J Urol. 2006;32(3):316–21.

80. Bishoff JT, Lackland AFB, Basler JW, Teichman JM, Thompson IM. Endoscopic subcutaneous modified inguinal lymph node dissection (ESMIL) for squamous cell carcinoma of the penis. J Urol. 2003;169:78.

81. Sotelo R, Sanchez-Salas R, Clavijo R. Endoscopic inguinal lymph node dissection for penile carcinoma: the developing of a novel technique. World J Urol. 2009;27(2):213–9.

82. Sotelo R, Sanchez-Salas R, Carmona O, Garcia A, Mariano M, Neiva G, et al. Endoscopic lymphadenectomy for penile carcinoma. J Endourol. 2007; 21(4):364–7. discussion 7.

83. Bevan-Thomas R, Slaton JW, Pettaway CA. Contemporary morbidity from lymphadenectomy for penile squamous cell carcinoma: the M.D. Anderson Cancer Center Experience. J Urol. 2002;167(4):1638–42.

84. Nelson BA, Cookson MS, Smith Jr JA, Chang SS. Complications of inguinal and pelvic lymphadenectomy for squamous cell carcinoma of the penis: a contemporary series. J Urol. 2004;172(2):494–7.

85. Jacobellis U. Modified radical inguinal lymphadenectomy for carcinoma of the penis: technique and results. J Urol. 2003;169(4):1349–52.

86. Parra RO. Accurate staging of carcinoma of the penis in men with nonpalpable inguinal lymph nodes by modified inguinal lymphadenectomy. J Urol. 1996; 155(2):560–3.

87. Ayyappan K, Ananthakrishnan N, Sankaran V. Can regional lymph node involvement be predicted in patients with carcinoma of the penis? Br J Urol. 1994;73(5):549–53.

88. Ornellas AA, Kinchin EW, Nobrega BL, Wisnescky A, Koifman N, Quirino R. Surgical treatment of invasive squamous cell carcinoma of the penis: Brazilian National Cancer Institute long-term experience. J Surg Oncol. 2008;97(6):487–95.

89. d'Ancona CA, de Lucena RG, Querne FA, Martins MH, Denardi F, Netto Jr NR. Long-term followup of

penile carcinoma treated with penectomy and bilateral modified inguinal lymphadenectomy. J Urol. 2004;172(2):498–501. discussion.

90. Coblentz TR, Theodorescu D. Morbidity of modified prophylactic inguinal lymphadenectomy for squamous cell carcinoma of the penis. J Urol. 2002;168(4 Pt 1): 1386–9.

91. Ettema HB, Kollen BJ, Verheyen CC, Buller HR. Prevention of venous thromboembolism in patients with immobilization of the lower extremities: a meta-analysis of randomized controlled trials. J Thromb Haemost. 2008;6(7):1093–8.

92. Sawczuk IS, Williams D, Chang DT. Low molecular weight heparin for venous thromboembolism prophylaxis in urologic oncologic surgery. Cancer Invest. 2002;20(7–8):889–92.

93. Horenblas S. Lymphadenectomy for squamous cell carcinoma of the penis. Part 2: the role and technique of lymph node dissection. BJU Int. 2001;88(5): 473–83.

94. Darouiche RO, Wall Jr MJ, Itani KM, Otterson MF, Webb AL, Carrick MM, et al. Chlorhexidine-alcohol versus povidone-iodine for surgical-site antisepsis. N Engl J Med. 2010;362(1):18–26.

95. Gallo Rolania FJ, Beneitez Alvarez ME, Izquierdo Garcia FM. The role of inguinal lymphadenectomy in epidermoid carcinoma of the penis. Use of Ligasure and analysis of the results. Arch Esp Urol. 2002;55(5):535–8.

96. Orefice S, Conti AR, Grassi M, Salvadori B. The use of lympho-venous anastomoses to prevent complications from ilio-inguinal dissection. Tumori. 1988; 74(3):347–51.

97. Bare RL, Assimos DG, McCullough DL, Smith DP, DeFranzo AJ, Marks MW. Inguinal lymphadenectomy and primary groin reconstruction using rectus abdominis muscle flaps in patients with penile cancer. Urology. 1994;44(4):557–61.

98. Tabatabaei S, McDougal WS. Primary skin closure of large groin defects after inguinal lymphadenectomy for penile cancer using an abdominal cutaneous advancement flap. J Urol. 2003;169(1):118–20.

99. Graafland NM, Moonen LM, van Boven HH, van Werkhoven E, Kerst JM, Horenblas S. Inguinal recurrence following therapeutic lymphadenectomy for node positive penile carcinoma: outcome and implications for management. J Urol. 2011;185(3): 888–93.

Rosa S. Djajadiningrat, René Sotelo,
Rafael Sanchez-Salas, Rafael Clavijo,
and Simon Horenblas

Introduction

The vast majority of penile cancers are squamous cell carcinomas (~95%). This subtype typically has a lymphatic drainage pattern. The presence of nodal involvement is the single most important prognostic factor [1–7]. The first draining lymph nodes (the "first-echelon" or "sentinel" nodes) are invariably within the inguinal lymphatic region. Thereafter, dissemination is to the pelvic nodes and/or distant sites. At initial presentation, distant metastases are present in only 1–2% of patients. Generally, patients with distant metastasis have also clinical evidence of (at least) inguinal nodal involvement [8]. Primary hematogenous spread has only been seen in sarcomatoid subtypes only [9]. Therefore, preoperative staging focuses primarily on the locoregional situation.

R.S. Djajadiningrat, M.D. (✉) • S. Horenblas, M.D., Ph.D.
Department of Urologic Oncology, Antoni van
Leeuwenhoek Hospital, The Netherlands Cancer
Institute, Plesmanlaan 121, Amsterdam 1066, CX,
The Netherlands
e-mail: s.horenblas@nki.nl

R. Sotelo, M.D.
Department of Urology, Instituto Médico La Floresta,
Caracas, Venezuela

R. Sanchez-Salas, M.D.
Department of Urology, Institut Mutualiste Monsouris,
Paris, France

R. Clavijo, M.D.
Department of Urology, Hospital de San Jose,
Bogota, Colombia

There is no controversy about the need for lymphadenectomy in patients with clinical evident nodal involvement. However, the optimal management of clinically node-negative (cN0) patients is subject of debate, since noninvasive staging techniques are limited in detecting small metastatic deposits. Approximately 20–25% of these cN0 patients have occult metastasis [10]. Current imaging techniques such as ultrasound, computed tomography (CT) and positron emission tomography (PET), as well as risk prediction based on primary tumor characteristics, have so far been unable to identify cN0 patients with occult metastases within reasonable limits [11–13].

Removal of nodal metastases at the earliest possible time, preferably in patients with impalpable lymph nodes and microscopic invasion only, improves survival considerably compared with surgical removal at the time when metastases become clinically apparent [9]. Some clinicians manage these cN0 patients with close surveillance, while others treat them with an elective inguinal node dissection based upon "risk-adapted approaches" [14]. While the former may lead to unintentional delay because of outgrowth of occult metastases in 20–25% of cN0 patients, the latter results in unnecessary lymph node dissection in 75–80% of cases, because of absence of metastasis [15]. Moreover, inguinal lymphadenectomy is associated with a high morbidity rate. Up to 35–70% of patients have short- or long-term complications [16–19].

Sentinel lymph node biopsy is a fairly new technique in medical practice that is becoming the standard of care for regional lymph node staging of many solid tumors. This technique is based on the hypothesis of stepwise distribution of malignant cells in the lymphatic system. The absence of tumor cells in the first lymph node(s) in the lymphatic drainage of the tumor indicates the absence of further spread in regional lymph node basin(s).

Sentinel lymph node biopsy is the preferred method of lymph node staging in melanoma and breast cancer [20]. This procedure has been included in the 2009 European Association of Urology guidelines on penile cancer [21].

Lymphatic Drainage of the Penis

The primary drainage of penile carcinoma is to the lymph nodes in the groin, and secondary drainage is to the lymph nodes in the pelvis. Bilateral inguinal drainage is considered the normal lymphatic anatomy of the penis. Lymphoscintigraphic studies in penile carcinoma have shown bilateral drainage in over 90% of patients [22]. The anatomy of the inguinal nodes has been described by various authors [23–25]. It is customary to divide inguinal nodes into two groups, superficial and deep. The superficial nodes are located beneath Scarpa's fascia and above the fascia lata covering the muscles of the thigh; around 8–25 nodes are present. There are three to five deep inguinal lymph nodes and these are situated around the fossa ovalis, the opening in the fascia lata where the saphenous vein drains into the femoral vein. The deep inguinal nodes connect the superficial nodes to the pelvic nodes. The deep inguinal nodes receive their afferents from the superficial nodes and directly from the deeper structures of the penis. The distinction of superficial and deep inguinal lymph nodes is clinically irrelevant since physical examination (palpation) cannot discern these anatomical entities from each other [26].

The so-called node of Cloquet or Rosenmüller is the most constant and usually largest inguinal node, located just underneath the inguinal ligament and medially to the femoral vein. Daseler et al. divided the inguinal region into five sections by drawing a horizontal and vertical line through the point where the saphenous vein drains into the femoral vein with one central zone directly overlying the junction [27]. With some individual variation, the nodes that are most frequently involved in penile carcinoma are typically located in Daseler's superiomedial section [28]. Skip metastases, circumventing the inguinal lymphatic region, to the pelvic lymph nodes are extremely rare and probably anecdotal [29, 30].

The pelvic nodes are located around the iliac vessels and in the obturator fossa, approximately 12–20. Inguinal lymphadenectomy consists of the removal of all regional nodes in the groin, and pelvic lymphadenectomy comprises the removal of all pelvic nodes.

Staging of Inguinal Lymph Nodes Using Dynamic Sentinel Node Biopsy

History

The sentinel lymph node concept was first described in parotid carcinomas by Gould and colleagues in 1960 [31]. Cabañas and coworkers investigated the sentinel lymph node concept in 46 cases of penile carcinoma in 1977. They injected contrast medium into the dorsal lymphatics of the penis and found "evidence of the existence of a specific lymph center, the so-called 'sentinel node,' in the lymphatic of the penis" [32].

It was assumed that a tumor-negative sentinel node was indicative for absence of further lymphatic spread and therefore no lymphadenectomy was anymore indicated. Sentinel node surgery consisted of identification and removal of this lymph node with completion lymphadenectomy only in those with a tumor-positive node. However, this initial "static" procedure, based on anatomic landmarks only, did not take into account individual drainage patterns. Several false-negative results were reported, and the technique was largely abandoned.

Reports of sentinel node biopsy in patients with breast cancer emerged in the 1990s, along with the development of alternative methods for identification of the sentinel node [33]. The sentinel node procedure was revived by Morton et al. in 1992, by using patent blue-V or isosulfan blue dye as a tracer enabling individual lymphatic mapping [34]. These methods, including the use of radioactive tracers and patent blue dye, were further investigated in cervical cancer, endometrial cancer, melanoma, and penile cancer [35–37]. Modern sentinel node biopsy is based on preoperative and perioperative imaging. Using a radioactive tracer, single photon emission computed tomography/computed tomography (SPECT/CT) scanning, patent blue during the operation, and a handheld gamma camera, the node labeled as the sentinel node can be found with greater accuracy.

Since 1994, DSNB has been performed at the authors' institution to stage cN0-patients [38].

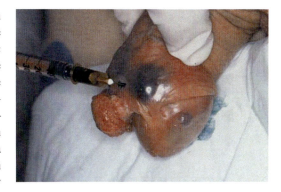

Fig. 7.1   Blue injection before surgery

Definition of a Sentinel Node

Which node can be defined as a sentinel node? The best definition is probably that of Morton: "the first lymph node that receives afferent drainage from a primary tumor" [39]. Early experiences in finding the sentinel node were hampered by high false-negative findings resulting from the individual variations in the anatomy of lymphatic drainage. With the advent of radioactive tracers, preoperative individual mapping of the lymphatic drainage became a reality. Tracing the sentinel node is currently possible with greater accuracy using preoperative lymphoscintigraphy and a handheld gamma detector during the operation to identify hot spots. Injecting patent blue just before surgery colors lymph channels and lymph nodes, helping the surgeon to identify the sentinel node and to distinguish second-echelon nodes from the sentinel node (Figs. 7.1 and 7.2). A hot spot in the inguinal region on the scintigram is considered a sentinel node if an afferent lymphatic channel is visualized, if the hot spot is the only one in the basin, or if the hot spot is seen in a sequential pattern. The location of the sentinel node is marked on the skin using real-time imaging and a [57]Co pen.

It is important to realize, that there is individual variation in the location of the sentinel node.

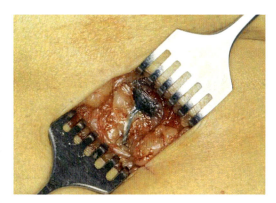

Fig. 7.2   Blue lymph channels and lymph nodes

Moreover, although the location is usually in the area traditionally known as the regional lymph node basin, aberrant locations can be seen in a minority of patients. Also more than one sentinel node can be present. All these variations can only be found if one combines all the preoperative information from the lymphoscintigraphy with the findings during surgery.

Lymphoscintigraphy

To localize the sentinel node preoperatively, lymphoscintigraphy is usually performed after intradermal peritumoral injection of colloid particles labeled with technetium-99m. The tracer is transported through the lymphatic channels to the first draining nodes in the groin and made visible on the lymphoscintigram as a "hot spot" (Fig. 7.3a). Lymph node uptake is based on

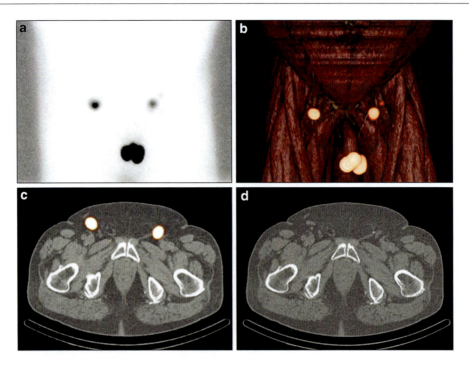

Fig. 7.3 (**a**) First draining nodes in the groin. Lymphoscintigram "hot spot." (**b–d**) SPECT-CT images after radioactive tracer injection

the ingestion of the colloid particles by the macrophages. Lymphoscintigraphy is usually performed the day or morning before surgery.

There are various reasons for using lymphoscintigraphy in the sentinel node procedure: to point out the draining lymph node field at risk for metastatic disease, to indicate the number of sentinel nodes, to distinguish first-echelon nodes from second echelon nodes, to identify lymph nodes in unpredictable locations and to mark the location of a sentinel node on the skin.

In European countries the most used tracer is technetium-99m nanocolloid with a particle size less than 80 nm. Typically, a dose of about 80 MBq is administered. It is strongly recommended to apply a spray containing 10% xylocaine or a local anesthetic cream at the injection site 30 min before tracer administration. This local anesthesia ensures that subsequent tracer injections are well tolerated and relatively easy to perform. A volume of 0.3 mL tracer fluid is subsequently administered intradermally around the tumor in three depots of 0.1 mL. Each depot is injected, raising a wheal. The tracer is injected

proximally of the tumor. For large tumors not restricted to the glans, the tracer can be administered in the retract prepuce or shaft. Injection margins within 1 cm of the primary tumor are recommended. In patients who have undergone previous excision, the injections may be administered around the scar using the same margins. Images are produced using a gamma camera with low-energy, high-resolution collimator.

Sentinel node lymphoscintigraphy must be sequential with images obtained at various time intervals. It should follow the sentinel lymph node concept, visualizing the lymphatic channels and identifying the lymph nodes receiving direct drainage from the tumor. To detect these lymph nodes, gamma camera acquisition consists of two parts: dynamic and static acquisition. After injection of the tracer, dynamic acquisition will be started for a period of 20 min to study the lymphatic flow. Subsequently, anterior and lateral static views will be obtained using a flood source to facilitate orientation. Static images will be repeated after 30 min and 2 h. Guided by the imaging, the location of the sentinel node is marked on the skin to enable perioperative localization using the handheld gamma ray detection probe, usually the following day [40].

Lymphoscintigraphy has been shown to be a very reproducible mode of imaging. In a study of 20 patients, two separate lymphoscintigrams were made and compared. There was virtually 100% concordance between the two studies [41]. Recently, hybrid SPECT-CT scanners have become available, allowing for the mapping of lymphatic drainage, after injection with a radioactive tracer, with unprecedented detail and in relation to anatomical landmarks obtained from the CT images (Fig. 7.3b–d).

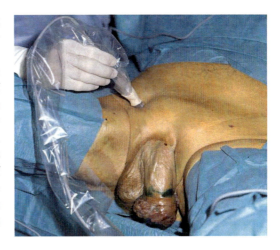

Fig. 7.4 Intraoperative sentinel node detection guided by the *blue* dye, a portable gamma camera and a gamma probe

Patent Blue

Perioperatively, patent blue dye can visualize lymphatic vessels and helps to differentiate sentinel nodes from second-echelon nodes. However, the use of blue dye alone is insufficient to reliably detect sentinel nodes. Differences between lymphatic mapping with radio labeled colloid and blue dye occur fairly often [37, 42, 43]. The two lymphatic mapping techniques are complementary. If only blue dye was used, almost 30% of the sentinel nodes would have been missed, because almost all harvested sentinel nodes were hot, whereas only about 70% were blue as well.

This may be caused by differences in the characteristics of the two tracers, the site of injection, or the difference in injected volume. In general, different physicians administer the radio labeled colloid and the blue dye independently and this may result in differences in injection technique and possible injection sites.

Identification of Sentinel Nodes

Bilateral drainage is seen in most patients. In the original description of Cabañas, this was seen in only 12% of patients [32]. Based on lymphoscintigraphic imaging, lymphatic drainage to both groins is seen in 80% of patients, unilateral drainage in 18%, and no drainage in

2% [44]. A mean number of 1.3 sentinel nodes per groin is visualized. Visualization appears to depend on the administered tracer dose. For optimal results, it is important that the administered dose of activity is sufficient and at least 60 MBq [45].

Intraoperative sentinel node detection is guided by the blue dye, a portable gamma camera and a gamma probe (Fig. 7.4). The portable gamma camera (Sentinella, Oncovision, Valencia, Spain) is used to guide the skin incisions and to obtain an intraoperative real-time visualization which allows detection of the sentinel nodes (Fig. 7.5). Then, the sentinel nodes are being traced using the acoustic guidance provided by a gamma ray detection probe (Neoprobe, Johnson & Johnson Medical, Germany). After excision of all preoperatively defined sentinel nodes, it is important to carefully search for any residual radioactivity using the probe to prevent that any remaining/additional sentinel nodes are left behind. Also images from the portable gamma camera can confirm removal of the sentinel nodes.

An important point is that the tumor load in the lymph nodes may also play a role in nonvisualization. Blocking of afferent lymph vessels by tumor cells is known to divert the tracer to other nodes, so-called rerouting, one of the reasons of a false-negative procedure (Fig. 7.6) [46].

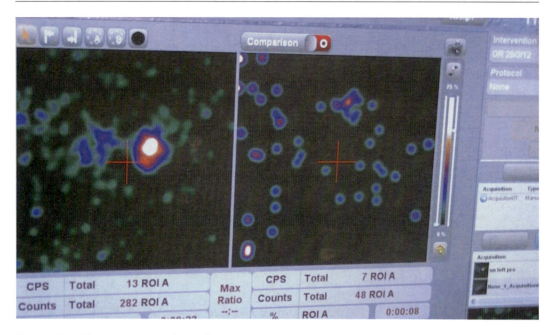

Fig. 7.5 Portable gamma camera (Sentinella, Oncovision, Valencia, Spain)

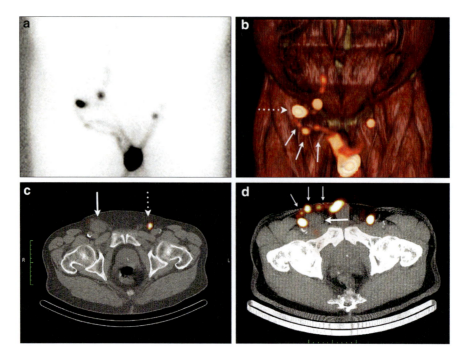

Fig. 7.6 Blocking of afferent lymph vessels by tumor cells diverting the tracer to other nodes, observed as a false-negative procedure

Reliability of Sentinel Node Procedure in Penis Cancer

Between 2000 and 2002, the early results of dynamic sentinel node biopsy (DSNB) in penile carcinoma were published [37, 40, 47]. Most sentinel nodes could be surgically identified with the aid of the tracer and the dye. Approximately 25% of patients had a tumor-positive sentinel node. Only these patients underwent additional inguinal lymph node dissection. The morbidity was limited, but the reliability of the procedure was not satisfactory because a false-negative rate of 22% was initially reported. Because the success of this novel procedure is determined by the false-negative rate, the false-negative cases were evaluated [42]. This analysis led to the following findings and adaptations. Non-visualized nodes were not explored in the early experience. Currently a second tracer injection is given in an attempt to find radioactive uptake and groins are always explored irrespective of the findings of the lymphoscintigram. Exploration of the groin after injection of the blue dye may still reveal a blue vessel leading to a nonradioactive sentinel node. Next to that, DSNB is also performed in patients with T1G2 en T1G3 tumors. Until 2004 patients with T1 tumors were managed with close surveillance and subsequent lymphadenectomy when metastases became clinically apparent. Also an additional SPECT/CT is made to visualize the anatomical location of the sentinel nodes [28].

Furthermore, micrometastases were missed initially; therefore, additional serial sectioning and immunohistochemical staining of the sentinel node with pankeratine and CAM 5.2 was added to standard hematoxylin and eosin staining.

Another cause of failure to find the sentinel node is blockage of inflow and rerouting of lymph caused by gross tumor involvement of the sentinel node. The true sentinel node is bypassed and the tracers are diverted to another node that is falsely labeled as the sentinel node. Rerouting was demonstrated on lymphoscintigrams and shown in patients with clinically involved nodes [46].

Therefore, high-resolution ultrasonography with fine-needle aspiration cytology (US-guided FNAC) was added as a routine examination before patients are scheduled for DSNB. Gross involvement of the sentinel node and tumor blocking might be picked up by US. Next to that, intraoperative palpation of the wound after sentinel node excision was appended to our protocol in order to identify suspicious nodes that failed to pick up any tracer.

A possible third cause of failure might be that the tumor cells are still in transit from the primary tumor to their landing zone at the time of the sentinel node biopsy. We know how fast lymph fluid travels through a lymph vessel, but little is known about the kinetics of tumor cells in lymphatics. Possibly, these unknown physiological factors are partially of influence in false-negative procedures [48].

One criticism has been the issue of the learning curve and the experience of the surgeon. Although experience is by all means important, the sentinel node biopsy is not considered major surgery. The issue of the learning curve was analyzed in a study by Leijte et al. who compared an experienced center with another center that only recently started with sentinel node biopsy. In a comparison of their first 30 patients, no difference between the two hospitals was noted [44].

Recently, a meta-analysis was performed on the issue of sentinel node biopsy of the penis. The authors concluded that this is a reliable procedure able to identify the sentinel node with high accuracy and a low number of false-negative findings (8%), especially if blue dye and radiotracer is used together. This is low enough to be considered safe and is comparable to recommendations for breast cancer patients (sensitivity 92%, specificity 100%) [49]. A two-center study including 592 explored groins showed a complication rate of only 4.7%, substantially lower than the reported complication rates of 35–70% in lymphadenectomy. The complications included wound infection, seroma/lymphocele, mild lymph edema, wound edge necrosis, and delayed bleeding [44].

Current research is focused on better visualization of the sentinel nodes using fluorescent dyes and a fluorescence camera. First results using a combination of radioactive tracers together with a fluorescence dye are promising, but further confirmation is mandatory [50].

Better imaging modalities are to be expected, although the promise of MR imaging with lymphotrophic nanoparticles (LN-MRI, ultrasmall particles of iron oxide, USPIOs, ferrumoxtran-10) has not been fulfilled yet, after showing promising results in identifying occult metastases in a study with penile cancer [51]. Unfortunately, ferrumoxtran-10 is not FDA-approved; hence it is not commercially available.

Rational for an Endoscopic Surgical Approach to Inguinal Lymph Nodes

Cost-benefit relation is hard to define in inguinal dissection for penile carcinoma. The dramatic wound-related complications have bound the procedure to a high morbidity rate. To provide a safe and oncologically sound dissection of the inguinal area while avoiding the dramatic consequences of wound dehiscence is the aim of the minimally invasive surgical approach to penile cancer. In our experience, in order to achieve surgical proficiency, inguinal dissection was initially planned and undertaken in a cadaveric model (Fig. 7.7). The useful applications of experimental models in urological surgery have been previously described [52].

Mathevet et al. [53] have presented an interesting experience with a gas-less endoscopic approach to inguinal dissection in vulvar and distal vaginal carcinoma. This is probably the most extensive experience for the inguinal endoscopic approach, and they reported low morbidity

outcomes with a single operative vascular lesion. They reported a 25% of perioperative complication rate, represented by lymphoceles observed in seven patients. In the urological field, Bishoff et al. [54] presented the initial experience with inguinal endoscopic dissection for penile carcinoma; they described a subcutaneous modified inguinal lymphadenectomy in two cadaveric models and in one patient with stage T3N1M0 penile carcinoma. This initial experience was not totally completed due to the presence of a large lymph node that precluded the dissection.

Tobias-Machado et al. reported a clinical experience with their video endoscopic inguinal lymphadenectomy (VEIL) technique; they described a series in which patients were submitted to classic open surgery in one limb and VEIL procedure in the contralateral member. All patients had non-palpable inguinal nodes and an indication for a bilateral procedure was based on the presence of risk factors for lymph node dissemination [55]. Our group has previously described a standardized technique of endoscopic groin dissection for penile carcinoma with a preoperative Doppler ultrasound mapping of the inguinal region [56]. More recently, Josephson et al. reported a robotic-assisted endoscopic inguinal lymphadenectomy in a 37 years old patient with palpable inguinal nodes despite oral antibiotics, with the authors proposing that robotic technology allows for three-dimensional optics, improved magnification, and an ergonomic platform, allowing for greater precision, dexterity, and degrees of freedom than that attainable using standard laparoscopic instruments [57].

Tobias–Machado et al. described in 2011 their initial experience with single-site VEIL in a 45-year-old man with pT2 grade 2 squamous cell penile carcinoma and impalpable inguinal nodes comparing VEIL with saphenous vein preservation in the left leg and single-site VEIL on the other side. No evidence of recurrence or port site metastasis were observed at 9 months of follow-up and the patient preferred the aesthetic result of the new technique described, with no complications were reported. Long-term studies are needed to truly evaluate the oncologic merit of

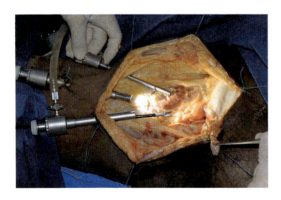

Fig. 7.7 Trocar placement verification on cadaver model this approach [58].

Patient Selection

Patients selected for endoscopic lymphadenectomy should be from a homogeneous patient population following the same principles of the open procedure: patients with palpable nodes, and patients without palpable nodes and a primary tumor with T2 high-grade cancer and/or vascular invasion [59]. Patients with palpable inguinal nodes should receive a 4–6 week course of antibiotic therapy, because 50% of initially positive nodes have an inflammatory etiology or a confirmatory percutaneous fine needle aspiration/biopsy of the inguinal mass to confirm its metastatic etiology.

Tailoring of therapeutics is an important issue in surgical treatment; in this matter we believe that intraoperative frozen section aids in the determination of a possible metastatic spread and therefore could suggest a more aggressive procedure. Frozen section has been incorporated into our surgical strategy.

It remains essential to remember that the selection of patients with no clinically positive inguinal disease for a prophylactic lymphadenectomy should be dictated by the pathologic characteristics of the primary penile tumor (i.e., stage, grade of primary tumor, and presence or absence of lymphovascular invasion) [4].

Surgical Technique

The endoscopic series are generally based on the surgical principles proposed by Catalona et al. [60]: a modified inguinal dissection with thicker skin flaps and preservation of the saphenous vein, which has been verified as an effective and oncologically safe procedure [61]. The VEIL technique does not spare the saphenous vein. In our experience, saphenous sparing was tailored based on operative findings; we believe that venous preservation would add to the avoidance of lymphocele, as well as an effective sealing of lymph vessels, and that is our rationale to deploy ultrasonic coagulation as part of the surgical procedure.

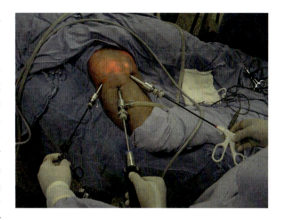

Fig. 7.8 Port placement and creation of working space

Mimicking open surgery, the dissection of superficial and deep inguinal node groups is undertaken. The anatomic boundaries that define the extension are the Sartorius muscle (lateral border), the adductor longus muscle (medial border), and the inguinal ligament and spermatic cord (superior border).

1. *Positioning and preparation.* Patients are positioned supine, one leg abducted with some knee flexion. Surgeon must be standing ipsilateral to the side where the lymphadenectomy is indicated, facing the upper side of the patient. The monitor is in the contralateral side. Surgeon and assistant must switch places during the procedure.

2. *Port placement and creation of working space.* The first incision is placed just below the apex of the femoral triangle in a medial position. Digital dissection is used to create space for a 10 mm trocar. The subcutaneous tissue plane is then bluntly developed with the endoscope, guided by light transmitting through the overlying skin. The objective is to create a subcutaneous space superficial to Scarpa's fascia. This space is then expanded with CO_2 insufflation at a pressure of 15 mmHg. Two additional ports are then positioned proximally in the lateral and medial lines of the femoral triangle. These are both 5 mm ports. In our initial experience, we used 10 and 5 mm trocars placed according to the surgeon's right and left arms, respectively (Fig. 7.8).

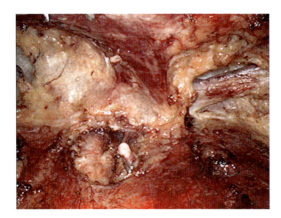

Fig. 7.9 Endoscopic inguinal surgical Weld (*right side*), sartorius muscle, adductor muscle, femoral artery, femoral vein, clipped saphenous vein, spermatic cord

3. *Initial dissection within the limits of the working space and identification of landmark structures.* The important landmark structures must be identified: the inguinal ligament, spermatic cord, femoral vessels, and saphenous vein. The lateral margin of the dissection is the sartorius muscle, the medial margin the adductor longus muscle, and the superior margin the inguinal ligament and spermatic cord (Fig. 7.9).

4. *Superficial component.* (a) Dissection of saphenous vein. The course of the saphenous vein is followed up to the saphenous arch at its junction with the superficial femoral vein. All lymph nodes identified along the saphenous vein and arch, as well as those identified in the path of the superficial epigastric vein should be removed. If possible and without compromising the dissection, veins draining to the saphenous arch and the saphenous vein itself should be spared. (b) Extraction of specimen. The nodal packet is placed in an impermeable sac and extracted. (c) Frozen section analysis of the superficial specimen. Initiation of the contralateral superficial dissection is conducted while awaiting the pathology results of the superficial dissection.

5. *Deep component.* The deep component of the lymphadenectomy is undertaken if frozen section results are positive for malignancy. (a) *Deep dissection.* Opening of the fascia lata and dissection along the medial side of femoral vein under the foramen ovalis up to the ingui-

nal ligament. Cloquet's node is to be identified beneath the inguinal ligament. (b) *Frozen section analysis of the deep specimen.* Depending on these results, laparoscopic pelvic lymphadenectomy may be indicated.

Frozen section analysis was performed in all cases of N0-2 disease before undertaking deep inguinal or pelvic lymphadenectomy. In one case, there was "fixed" nodal disease unilaterally that was approached in a standard open fashion. Thus, we summarize 14 procedures in eight patients. Positive frozen section analysis was the indication for deep dissection in three cases, and one node was retrieved from each of these dissections. The patient who underwent deep inguinal and pelvic lymph node dissection had enlarged iliac nodes on CT scan. Three lymph nodes were obtained from the pelvic dissection. Pelvic lymphadenectomy is performed from the bifurcation of the common iliac vessels distal to the passage of lymphatic nodes into the groin, medial to the genitofemoral nerve into the obturator fossa. A 10 mm trocar for the scope is placed at the umbilicus. Three other trocars are placed by the surgeon and/or assistant: one 5 mm pararectal trocar on each side and an additional 10 mm trocar in the iliac fossa on the surgeon's side. The limits of dissection are the same as those of an obturator and iliac pelvic lymph node dissection, but include the obturator fossa, as mentioned [62].

The saphenous vein and its branches were preserved in six groins. Saphenous vein sparing was not intended in patients with N2-3 disease. The final decision was based on the intra-operative surgical findings. Deep dissection was planned regardless of the frozen section results in all cases.

6. Drainage placement was achieved through the initial port site (Fig. 7.10).

7. Closure of all surgical incisions.

8. Placement of compression stockings immediately following the surgical procedure.

A special consideration with the endoscopic technique in the inguinal area encompasses the management of the CO_2 in the subcutaneous tissue. None of the published series have

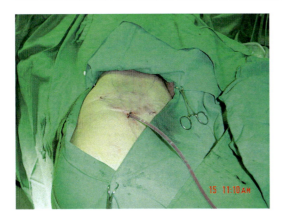

Fig. 7.10 Drainage placement

reported important complications regarding this specific issue. In the first case series, our anesthesia team claimed concern in the possibility of an augmented systemic absorption of CO_2 from this endoscopic approach. In this regard, we pay careful attention to frequent evacuation of the gas insufflation at the completion of the surgical procedure, in order to avoid gas absorption of gas within the surrounding tissues. Furthermore, we intend to limit gas expansion in the subcutaneous tissue with the use of elastic drapes placed both cranial and cephalad to the inguinal area being surgically explored.

Saphenous Vein Sparing and Deployment of Ultrasonic Coagulation

Our rationale for saphenous vein sparing is that lymphoceles are often caused by removal of lymph nodes and the resulting dysfunction/disruption in the lymph carrying channels. The remaining saphenous vein would aid in rerouting the lower limb lymph fluid. Regarding ultrasonic coagulation, an effective sealing of the lymph vessels in inguinal lymphadenectomy has been previously described with the use of thermal energy [63]. Furthermore, Kajiyama et al. presented a comparative study in which they verify the sealing of the thoracic duct by using

ultrasonic coagulating shears. They compared bursting pressure of the thoracic duct and left gastric artery within surgical specimens. The mean bursting pressure of the thoracic duct was high enough to support the clinical use of this device, and was significantly higher than that of the left gastric artery [64]. Ohtsuka et al. [65] have reported their clinical experience using ultrasonic shears which could effectively seal lymphatics. They successfully used the harmonic scalpel to obliterate the thoracic duct in cases of chylous ascites. The latter constitutes our rationale to advice deployment of ultrasonic shears in our endoscopic procedures. On the other hand, a clinical trial in breast cancer presented by Adwani and Ebbs [66] showed no benefit of the ultrasonic shears over standard coagulation techniques in decreasing seroma formation, and thus the issue remains somewhat controversial.

Cancer Control

The true measure of the quality of a lymphadenectomy procedure is objectively measured via the number of lymph nodes harvested at the time of the procedure [67]. It is estimated 8–25 superficial nodes are present above the fascia lata and beneath the subcutaneous fascia [9]. Lont et al. reported a range between 3 and 20 inguinal lymph nodes resected utilizing an open surgical approach [68].

For the novel endoscopic approach, the number numbers of nodes retrieved have ranged between 9 and 10 in published series [56, 69]. Tobias-Machado et al. did not report increased rates of recurrence or disease progression using an endoscopic approach. It is novel that in this series both a VEIL and classic open approach were compared, and simultaneously performed in the same patient. However, their updated series with 10 patients at a mean follow-up of 18.7 months (range 12–31) report no signs of recurrence or disease progression, which is very encouraging [69]. More recently, Tobias-Machado and colleagues reassessed their clinical experience with the VEIL approach and presented a comparative study. Twenty limbs underwent VEIL and ten-limbs underwent an open procedure. Mean operative time was 120 min for VEIL and 92 min for the open procedure. There was no difference in the number of nodes removed or in the incidence of positive lymph nodes for metastases. They observed complications in 70% and 20% of limbs that underwent open and endoscopic surgery, respectively. At a median follow-up period of 33 months, they have not observed any recurrences [70].

We have reported a unilateral inguinal recurrence in one patient at a follow-up of 1 year. We acknowledge that this recurrence was found in a patient with fixed nodal disease unilaterally who was likely not the most suitable candidate for this endoscopic approach.

The oncological results from published series are alike, even when they are contrasted across different patient cohorts. Tobias-Machado et al. [70] performed mostly prophylactic inguinal lymphadenectomies and Sotelo et al. [56] performed the procedure in patients with palpable lymph nodes. Robot-assisted experience reported an average operative time of 125 min, estimated blood losses of 75 cc, and an estimated 11 superficial and eight deep inguinal lymph nodes extracted with no complications described [71].

Recently, Alnajiar et al. described extracapsular spread (ECS) of tumor in inguinal lymph nodes as an independent prognosticator of survival reporting that in 411 patients, extensive and multifocal inguinal ECS portend poorer survival rates and cancer-specific outcomes. Thirty-nine patients with ECS were identified over a 10-year period, with 5-year cancer-specific survival rates in patients with single node involvement (pN1) and ECS spread being 25% vs. 100% without ECS and in patients with multiple/bilateral node involvement (pN2) with ECS 27% vs. 81.5% without ECS. The 5-year cancer-specific survival with focal ECS is 47%, extensive ECS 27.5%, and multifocal ECS 0%. Hence, it is evident such patients should be under close surveillance and chemotherapy should be considered in the early adjuvant setting [72].

Complications and Morbidity

Lymphadenectomy is associated with significant morbidity (24–87%) like wound infection, skin necrosis, subcutaneous seroma, and lymphedema [73]. Despite the small number of patients treated and only short to intermediate follow-up available, there is a decrease in cutaneous complications and a trend toward decreased overall morbidity with an endoscopic approach [55, 56]. Similarly, no intraoperative complications have been reported in these endoscopic series.

In the field of penile cancer, there are certain unanswered and highly debated controversies such as should a bilateral inguinal lymph node dissection be performed in all patients with only unilateral palpable nodes? Should a prophylactic inguinal lymphadenectomy be the preferred approach in patients with no clinically evident inguinal lymphadenopathy? What are the specific indications (if any) for performing a pelvic lymphadenectomy? The concern of perioperative morbidity remains a cornerstone in our decision tree which pertain as to how can we optimize the care of penile cancer.

Discussion

As reported by Lont et al. the treatment of inguinal metastases has evolved across most international cancer referral centers in recent years; 85 patients with primary T2-3N0M0 penile cancer patients with non-palpable inguinal lymph nodes were treated with surveillance and then compared with 68 patients with similar clinical characteristics whom underwent DSNB. Disease specific 3-year survival in the surveillance vs. sentinel node groups was 79% and 91%, respectively [74]. More recently, immediate lymphadenectomy was indicated for invasive and high-risk primary penile tumors and as previously described, novel techniques have been applied to our surgical armamentarium [11, 37, 38]. Banerjee et al. concluded that dynamic sentinel lymph node biopsy at the time of primary surgery is both minimally invasive and accurate. Similarly, it does not have the morbidity of lymphadenectomy and the risks inherent to a general anesthesia in addition to obviating the need for further surgery. These authors showed in a series of 39 patients that there were no false negative results for the 16 patients that required lymph node surgery by adopting this approach in patients with primary tumor histology pT1G2 or greater squamous cell carcinoma of the penis with clinically node-negative (cN0) [75].

Minimally invasive surgery within the field of urology has flourished over the past two decades with outstanding results. This approach has not only proven its feasibility in many subspecialties of urology but also preserved the surgical principles of open surgery. More recently, laparoscopy has come forward in the field of reconstructive urologic surgery and laparoscopic surgeons have reproduced the traditional operations in the endoscopic surgical environment maintaining comparable results [76]. Endoscopic inguinal lymphadenectomy represents the evolution of a key oncologic surgical procedure in penile cancer. Although clinical experience is still limited with endoscopic inguinal lymph node dissection, it appears to have less wound-related morbidity and the early oncologic results are encouraging. Schwentner et al. presented in 2012, equivalence in terms of a cancer control endpoint comparing it to the open approach at a mean follow-up of 55.3 months (2–87); 60 procedures were performed and 26 were completed entirely endoscopically. The mean operative time for open lymphadenectomy (OL) was 101.7 min (38–195) which was significantly shorter than for endoscopic lymphadenectomy (EL) (136.3 min, 87–186), $p < 0.001$. Both groups were comparable with respect to the number of nodes harvested (OL 7.2, 2–16 vs. EL 6.9, 4–13) as well as to the number of positive lymph nodes (OL 1.8 vs. EL 1.6). Leg edema or secondary wound healing were extremely rare (1/26) after EL, with an overall complication rate of 7.7%. In contrast, complications occurred in more than half of the OL cases (55.3%). Rates of local recurrence and systemic cancer dissemination were identical in OL vs. EL [77]. The prognostic significance of ECS and its extent in inguinal nodes in penile cancer has been demonstrated by Alnajjar et al. whom once again reported that ECS within the inguinal lymphadenectomy specimen was an independent predictor of survival with patients exhibiting extensive and multifocal inguinal ECS having a significantly reduced survival rate and poorer outcome [78].

Greater experience and long-term follow-up are evidently required before adopting this as an acceptable alternative to the standard open inguinal lymph node dissection.

The future care of penile cancer patients will probably integrate a therapeutic approach to avoid not only unnecessary surgery, but also adopt a surgical approach with the lowest risk of perioperative complications. The recently proven reliability and safety of DSNB will likely continue to play an important role in the management of penile cancer [79, 80], with lessons learned from breast cancer and melanoma serving as a preview on how this minimally invasive diagnostic and therapeutic approach will be utilized in our care of penile cancer patients. The inguinal endoscopic approach will likely as well be embraced as a mainstream approach to assessing and eradicating inguinal lymph node metastasis within this patient population.

Conclusion

Endoscopic Lymphadenectomy is still evolving as a surgical approach in the management of penile cancer, and it is evident that larger surgical series with long-term follow-up are needed before we can unequivocally integrate it as a first-line surgical approach to the management of inguinal lymph nodes among penile cancer patients. While penile cancer is a rare disease, we must never lose sight of its often highly aggressive natural history and current research should continue to pursue ways to decrease the morbidity inherent our therapeutic approaches while not compromising the oncologic outcomes.

References

1. Srinivas V, Morse MJ, Herr HW, Sogani PC, Whitmore WF. Penile cancer: relation of extent of nodal metastasis to survival. J Urol. 1987;137(5):880–2.
2. Ravi R. Correlation between the extent of nodal involvement and survival following groin dissection for carcinoma of the penis. Br J Urol. 1993;72(5 Pt 2): 817–9.
3. Horenblas S, Van Tinteren H, Delemarre JFM, Moonen LMF, Lustig V, van Waardenburg EW. Squamous cell carcinoma of the penis. III Treatment of regional lymph nodes. 1993;492–7.
4. Sánchez-Ortiz RF, Pettaway CA. The role of lymphadenectomy in penile cancer. Urologic Oncol. 2004;22(3):236–44. discussion 244–5.
5. Pandey D, Mahajan V, Kannan RR. Prognostic factors in node-positive carcinoma of the penis. J Surg Oncol. 2006;93(2):133–8.
6. Lont AP, Kroon BK, Gallee MPW, van Tinteren H, Moonen LMF, Horenblas S. Pelvic lymph node dissection for penile carcinoma: extent of inguinal lymph node involvement as an indicator for pelvic lymph node involvement and survival. J Urol. 2007;177(3):947–52. discussion 952.
7. Ornellas AA, Kinchin EW, Nóbrega BLB, Wisnescky A, Koifman N, Quirino R. Surgical treatment of invasive squamous cell carcinoma of the penis: Brazilian National Cancer Institute long-term experience. J Surg Oncol. 2008;97(6):487–95.
8. Culkin DJ, Beer TM. Advanced penile carcinoma. J Urol. 2003;170(2 Pt 1):359–65.
9. Kroon BK, Horenblas S, Lonta P, Tanis PJ, Gallee MPW, Nieweg OE. Patients with penile carcinoma benefit from immediate resection of clinically occult lymph node metastases. J Urol. 2005;173(3):816–9.
10. Abi-Aad AS, deKernion JB. Controversies in ilioinguinal lymphadenectomy for cancer of the penis. Urol Clin North Am. 1992;19(2):319–24.
11. Horenblas S, Van Tinteren H, Delemarre JF, Moonen LM, Lustig V, Kröger R. Squamous cell carcinoma of the penis: accuracy of tumor, nodes and metastasis classification system, and role of lymphangiography, computerized tomography scan and fine needle aspiration cytology. J Urol. 1991;146(5):1279–83.
12. Hegarty PK, Kayes O, Freeman A, Christopher N, Ralph DJ, Minhas S. A prospective study of 100 cases of penile cancer managed according to European Association of Urology guidelines. BJU Int. 2006;98(3):526–31.
13. Sadeghi R, Gholami H, Zakavi SR, Kakhki VRD, Horenblas S. Accuracy of 18F-FDG PET/CT for diagnosing inguinal lymph node involvement in penile squamous cell carcinoma. Clin Nucl Med. 2012;37: 436–41.
14. Solsona E, Algaba F, Horenblas S, Pizzocaro G, Windahl T. EAU guidelines on penile cancer. Eur Urol. 2004;46(1):1–8.
15. Ficarra V, Zattoni F, Cunico SC, Galetti TP, Luciani L, Fandella A, et al. Lymphatic and vascular embolizations are independent predictive variables of inguinal lymph node involvement in patients with squamous cell carcinoma of the penis: Gruppo Uro-Oncologico del Nord Est (Northeast Uro-Oncological Group) Penile Cancer Data Base data. Cancer. 2005;103(12):2507–16.
16. Johnson DE, Lo RK. Complications of groin dissection in penile cancer. Experience with 101 lymphadenectomies. Urology. 1984;24(4):312–4.
17. Ornellas AA, Seixas AL, de Moraes JR. Analyses of 200 lymphadenectomies in patients with penile carcinoma. J Urol. 1991;146(2):330–2.
18. Ravi R. Morbidity following groin dissection for penile carcinoma. Br J Urol. 1993;72(6):941–5.
19. Bevan-Thomas R, Slaton JW, Pettaway CA. Contemporary morbidity from lymphadenectomy for penile squamous cell carcinoma: the M.D. Anderson Cancer Center Experience. J Urol. 2002;167(4): 1638–42.
20. Berveiller P, Mir O, Veyrie N, Barranger E. The sentinel-node concept: a dramatic improvement in breast-cancer surgery. Lancet Oncol. 2010;11(9):906.
21. Pizzocaro G, Algaba F, Horenblas S, Solsona E, Van der Poel H, Watkin N. EAU penile cancer guidelines 2009. Eur Urol. 2010;57(6):1002–12.
22. Hadway P, Smith Y, Corbishley C, Heenan S, Watkin NA. Evaluation of dynamic lymphoscintigraphy and sentinel lymph-node biopsy for detecting occult metastases in patients with penile squamous cell carcinoma. BJU Int. 2007;100(3):561–5.
23. Cabanas R. Anatomy and biopsy of sentinel nodes. Urol Clin North Am. 1992;19(2):267–76.
24. Crawford ED, Daneshgari F. Management of regional lymphatic drainage in carcinoma of the penis. Urol Clin North Am. 1992;19(2):305–17.
25. Dewire D, Lepor H. Anatomic considerations of the penis and its lymphatic drainage. Urol Clin North Am. 1992;19:211–9.
26. Horenblas S. Lymphadenectomy for squamous cell carcinoma of the penis. Part 1: diagnosis of lymph node metastasis. BJU Int. 2001;88(5):467–72.
27. Daseler EH, Anson BJ, Reimann AF. Radical excision of the inguinal and iliac lymph glands; a study based upon 450 anatomical dissections and upon supportive clinical observations. Surg Gynecol Obstet. 1948; 87(6):679–94.
28. Leijte JA, Valdés Olmos RA, Nieweg OE, Horenblas S. Anatomical mapping of lymphatic drainage in penile carcinoma with SPECT-CT: implications for the extent of inguinal lymph node dissection. Eur Urol. 2008;54(4):885–90.
29. Lopes A, Bezerra AL, Serrano SV, Hidalgo GS. Iliac nodal metastases from carcinoma of the penis treated surgically. BJU Int. 2000;86(6):690–3.
30. Wood HM, Angermeier KW. Anatomic considerations of the penis, lymphatic drainage, and biopsy of the sentinel node. Urol Clin North Am. 2010;37(3):327–34.

31. Gould EA, Winship T, Philbin PH, Kerr HH. Observations on a "sentinel node" in cancer of the parotid. Cancer. 1960;13:77–8.

32. Cabanas R. An approach for the treatment of penile carcinoma. Cancer. 1977;39(2):456–66.

33. Veronesi U, Paganelli G, Galimberti V, Viale G, Zurrida S, Bedoni M, et al. Sentinel-node biopsy to avoid axillary dissection in breast cancer with clinically negative lymph-nodes. Lancet. 1997;349(9069):1864–7.

34. Morton DL, Wen DR, Wong JH, Economou JS, Cagle LA, Storm FK, et al. Technical details of intraoperative lymphatic mapping for early stage melanoma. Arch Surg (Chicago, IL: 1960). 1992;127(4):392–9.

35. De Cicco C, Cremonesi M, Luini A, Bartolomei M, Grana C, Prisco G, et al. Lymphoscintigraphy and radioguided biopsy of the sentinel axillary node in breast cancer. J Nucl Med: Official Publ Soc Nucl Med. 1998;39(12):2080–4.

36. Dale PS, Williams JT. Axillary staging utilizing selective sentinel lymphadenectomy for patients with invasive breast carcinoma. Am Surg. 1998;64(1):28–31. discussion 32.

37. Horenblas S, Jansen L, Meinhardt W, Hoefnagel CA, de Jong D, Nieweg OE. Detection of occult metastasis in squamous cell carcinoma of the penis using a dynamic sentinel node procedure. J Urol. 2000; 163(1):100–4.

38. Leijte JAP, Kroon BK, Valdés Olmos RA, Nieweg OE, Horenblas S. Reliability and safety of current dynamic sentinel node biopsy for penile carcinoma. Eur Urol. 2007;52(1):170–7.

39. Morton DL, Bostick PJ. Will the true sentinel node please stand? Ann Surg Oncol. 1999;6(1):12–4.

40. Valdés Olmos RA, Tanis PJ, Hoefnagel CA, Jansen L, Nieweg OE, Meinhardt W, et al. Penile lymphoscintigraphy for sentinel node identification. Eur J Nucl Med Mol Imaging. 2001;28(5):581–5.

41. Kroon BK, Valdés Olmos RA, van Tinteren H, Nieweg OE, Horenblas S. Reproducibility of lymphoscintigraphy for lymphatic mapping in patients with penile carcinoma. J Urol. 2005;174(6):2214–7.

42. Kroon BK, Horenblas S, Estourgie SH, Lont AP, Valdés Olmos RA, Nieweg OE. How to avoid false-negative dynamic sentinel node procedures in penile carcinoma. J Urol. 2004;171(2):663. author reply 663.

43. Kroon BK, Horenblas S, Meinhardt W, van der Poel HG, Bex A, van Tinteren H, et al. Dynamic sentinel node biopsy in penile carcinoma: evaluation of 10 years experience. Eur Urol. 2005;47(5):601–6. discussion 606.

44. Leijte JAP, Hughes B, Graafland NM, Kroon BK, Olmos RAV, Nieweg OE. et al. Two-center evaluation of dynamic sentinel node biopsy for squamous cell carcinoma of the penis. J Clin Oncol: Official J Am Soc Clin Oncol. 2009;27(20):3325–9.

45. Kroon BK, Valdés Olmos R, Nieweg OE, Horenblas S. Non-visualization of sentinel lymph nodes in penile carcinoma. Eur J Nucl Med Mol Imaging. 2005;32(9): 1096–9.

46. Leijte JAP, van der Ploeg IMC, Valdés Olmos RA, Nieweg OE, Horenblas S. Visualization of tumor blockage and rerouting of lymphatic drainage in penile cancer patients by use of SPECT/CT. J Nucl Med: Official Publ Soc Nucl Med. 2009;50(3): 364–7.

47. Tanis PJ, Lonta P, Meinhardt W, Olmos RAV, Nieweg OE, Horenblas S. Dynamic sentinel node biopsy for penile cancer: reliability of a staging technique. J Urol. 2002;168(1):76–80.

48. Nieweg OE. False-negative sentinel node biopsy. Ann Surg Oncol. 2009;16(8):2089–91.

49. Sadeghi R, Gholami H, Zakavi SR, Kakhki VRD, Tabasi KT, Horenblas S. Accuracy of sentinel lymph node biopsy for inguinal lymph node staging of penile squamous cell carcinoma: systematic review and meta-analysis of the literature. J Urol. 2012;187(1):25–31.

50. Brouwer O, Buckle T, Vermeeren L, Klop W, Balm A, van der Poel H, et al. Comparing the novel hybrid radioactive/fluorescent tracer ICG-99mTc-nanocolloid with 99mTc-nanocolloid for sentinel node identification: a validation study using lymphoscintigraphy and SPECT/CT. J Nucl Med. 2012;53(7):1034–40.

51. Tabatabaei S, Harisinghani M, McDougal WS. Regional lymph node staging using lymphotropic nanoparticle enhanced magnetic resonance imaging with ferumoxtran-10 in patients with penile cancer. J Urol. 2005;174(3):923–7. discussion 927.

52. van Velthoven RF, HoVmann P. Methods for laparoscopic training using animal models. Curr Urol Rep. 2006;7(2):114–9.

53. Mathevet P, Schettini S, Roy M, et al. Inguinoscopy or video-endoscopic lymph node dissection. The trocar. J Gynecol Surg Endosc. 2002. Jan 2nd (Online Video)

54. Bishoff JT, Basler JW, Teichman JM, et al. Endoscopic subcutaneous modified inguinal lymph node dissection (ESMIL) for squamous cell carcinoma of the penis. J Urol. 2003. (Abstract # 301)

55. Tobias-Machado M, Tavares A, Molina WR, et al. Video endoscopic inguinal lymphadenectomy (VEIL): minimally invasive resection of inguinal lymph nodes. Int Braz J Urol. 2006;32(3):316–21.

56. Sotelo R, Sánchez-Salas R, Carmona O, Garcia A, Mariano M, Neiva G, Trujillo G, Novoa J, Cornejo F, Finelli A. Endoscopic lymphadenectomy for penile carcinoma. J Endourol. 2007;21(4):364–7.

57. Josephson D, Jacobsohn K, Link B, Wilson T. Robotic-assisted endoscopic inguinal lymphadenectomy. Urology. 2009;73:167–71.

58. Tobias-Machado M, Correa W, Ries L, Starling E, Castro Neves O, Juliano R, Pompeo A. J Endourol. 2011;25(4):607–10.

59. Algaba F, Horenblas S, Pizzocaro Luigi Piva G, Solsona E, Windahl T. T urology EAo. EAU guidelines on penile cancer. Eur Urol. 2002;42(3):199–203.

60. Catalona WJ. A modified inguinal lymphadenectomy for carcinoma of the penis with preservation of saphenous veins: technique and preliminary results. J Urol. 1988;140:306–10.

61. Colberg JW, Andriole GL, Catalona WJ. Long-term follow-up of men undergoing modiWed inguinal lymphadenectomy for carcinoma of the penis. Br J Urol. 1997;79(1):54–7.

62. Assimos DG, Jarow JP. Role of laparoscopic pelvic lymph node dissection in the management of patients with penile cancer and inguinal adenopathy. J Endourol. 1994;8(5):365–9.

63. Gallo Rolania FJ, Beneitez Alvarez ME, Izquierdo García FM. The role of inguinal lymphadenectomy in epidermoid carcinoma of the penis. Use of Ligasure and analysis of the results. Arch Esp Urol. 2002;55(5):535–8.

64. Kajiyama Y, Iwanuma Y, Tomita N, Amano T, Hattori K, Tsurumaru M. Sealing the thoracic duct with ultrasonic coagulating shears. Hepatogastroenterology. 2005;52(64):1053–6.

65. Ohtsuka T, Nimomiya M, Kobayashi J, Kaneko Y. VATS thoracic-duct division for aortic surgery-related chylous leakage. Eur J Cardiothorac Surg. 2005;27(1):153–5.

66. Adwani A, Ebbs SR. Ultracision reduces acute blood loss but not seroma formation after mastectomy and axillary dissection: a pilot study. Int J Clin Pract. 2006;60(5):562–4.

67. Herr HW. The concept of lymph node density—is it ready for clinical practice? J Urol. 2007;177(4): 1273–5.

68. Lont AP, Kroon BK, Gallee MP, van Tinteren H, Moonen LM, Horenblas S. Pelvic lymph node dissection for penile carcinoma: extent of inguinal lymph node involvement as an indicator for pelvic lymph node involvement and survival. J Urol. 2007;177(3):947–52.

69. Tobias-Machado M, Tavares A, Ornellas AA, Molina Jr WR, Juliano RV, Wroclawski ER. Video endoscopic inguinal lymphadenectomy: a new minimally invasive procedure for radical management of inguinal nodes in patients with penile squamous cell carcinoma. J Urol. 2007;177(3):953–7.

70. Tobias-Machado M, Tavares A, Silva MN, Molina Jr WR, Forseto PH, Juliano RV, Wroclawski ER. Can video endoscopic inguinal lymphadenectomy achieve a lower morbidity than open lymph node dissection in penile cancer patients? J Endourol. 2008;22(8): 1687–91.

71. Josephson D, Jacobsohn K, Link B, Wilson T. Robotic-assisted endoscopic inguinal lymphadenectomy. Urology. 2009;73:167–71.

72. Alnajjar HM, Tinwell B, Rajab R, Kousparos G, Perry MJA, Corbishley CM, Watkin NA. Prognostic significance of extracapsular spread and its extent in inguinal nodes in penile cancer. Poster presented at: 27th Annual Congress of the European Association of Urology; 2012 Feb 24–28, Paris–France

73. Misra S, Chaturvedi A, Misra NC. Penile carcinoma: a challenge for the developing world. Lancet Oncol. 2004;5(4):240–7.

74. Banerjee S, Finch W, Rafiq M, Sethia KK, Kumar V. Dynamic sentinel lymph node biopsy at the time of primary surgery; impact on morbidity and outcome. Poster presented at: 27th Annual Congress of the European Association of Urology; 2012 Feb 24–28, Paris–France

75. Lont AP, Horenblas S, Tanis PJ, Gallee MP, van Tinteren H, Nieweg OE. Management of clinically node negative penile carcinoma: improved survival after the introduction of dynamic sentinel node biopsy. J Urol. 2003;170(3):783–6.

76. Kaouk JH, Gill IS. Laparoscopic reconstructive urology. J Urol. 2003;170:1070–3.

77. Schwentner C, Todenhöfer T, Schilling D, Aufderklamm S, Mundhenk J, Alloussi S, Gakis G. Endoscopic inguinofemoral lymphadenectomy for penile malignancies—extended follow-up. Poster presented at: 27th Annual Congress of the European Association of Urology; 2012 Feb 24–28, Paris–France

78. Alnajjar HM, Tinwell B, Rajab R, Kousparos G, Perry MJA, Corbishley CM, Watkin NA. Prognostic significance of extracapsular spread and its extent in inguinal nodes in penile cancer. Poster presented at: 27th Annual Congress of the European Association of Urology; 2012 Feb 24–28, Paris–France

79. Leijte JA, Kroon BK, Valdés Olmos RA, Nieweg OE, Horenblas S. Reliability and safety of current dynamic sentinel node biopsy for penile carcinoma. Eur Urol. 2007;52(1):170–7.

80. Spiess PE, Izawa JI, Bassett R, Kedar D, Busby JE, Wong F, Eddings T, Tamboli P, Pettaway CA. Preoperative lymphoscintigraphy and dynamic sentinel node biopsy for staging penile cancer: results with pathological correla. J Urol. 2007;177:2157–61.

Applications of Radiation Therapy in the Management of Penile Cancer

8

Juanita Crook and Matthew Biagioli

Introduction

Squamous carcinoma of the penis is a radiosensitive tumor that lends itself well to curative treatment by radiotherapy. Small tumors under 4 cm and limited to the glans and/or prepuce can be ideally managed with brachytherapy while larger more advanced tumors and those with nodal involvement are better managed with external beam radiotherapy (EBRT). Surgical salvage is reserved for local treatment failures. Successful treatment avoids penile amputation and is more readily achieved with brachytherapy than with EBRT. Ten-year penile sparing rates are reported at approximately 70% after brachytherapy while for more advanced tumors treated with EBRT penile sparing at 5 years is about 60%. Due to the unique anatomic features, specialized techniques are required; these are described in detail.

J. Crook, M.D. (✉)
Department of Radiation Oncology,
British Columbia Cancer Agency,
399, Royal Avenue, Kelowna, BC, Canada VIY 5L3
e-mail: jcrook@bccancer.bc.ca

M. Biagioli, M.D., M.S.
Department of Radiation Oncology,
H. Lee Moffitt Cancer Center, Tampa, FL, USA
e-mail: Matthew.Biagioli@moffitt.org

Anatomy and Lymph Drainage

The penis is composed of the corpus spongiosum and two corpora cavernosa bound together in Buck's fascia. The corpus spongiosum expands distally into the glans penis, which is covered by the prepuce (foreskin). The skin of the penis and prepuce drain primarily to the superficial inguinal nodes, especially the supero-medial zone where the sentinel node is located. The lymphatics of the glans drain to the superficial inguinal nodes or directly to the deep inguinal or even the external iliac group. The lymphatics of the corporal bodies drain to the superficial or deep inguinal nodes or directly to the external iliac nodes. From a surgical standpoint, the simultaneous removal of first- and second-echelon lymph nodes is traditionally called an ilioinguinal lymph node dissection (ILND).

Penile Cancer Management and Quality of Life

Management of carcinoma of the penis has traditionally been surgical resection, ranging from circumcision to conservative local excision, laser ablation, and Mohs micrographic surgery to the more morbid partial or total penectomy. Local failure rates range from 10 to 56% for conservative approaches and 0 to 18% for partial

P.E. Spiess (ed.), *Penile Cancer: Diagnosis and Treatment*, Current Clinical Urology,
DOI 10.1007/978-1-62703-367-1_8, © Springer Science+Business Media New York 2013

or total penectomy [1, 2]. However, since partial and total penectomy are associated with considerable psychological morbidity, the option of organ preservation should be discussed with all early-stage patients.

In a small study reported by Opjordsmoen et al., patients undergoing radiation therapy had better global sexual scores than those undergoing partial penectomy or local excision [3]. Maddineni et al. analyzed 128 patients from six studies of surgically managed penile carcinoma patients. Five contained retrospective data while one study collected prospective data on erectile function [4]. Two studies using the General Health Questionnaire (GHQ) showed impaired well-being in up to 40%, with the patients who underwent more mutilating treatments more likely to have impairment. Two used the Hospital Anxiety and Depression Score (HADS) and demonstrated pathological anxiety in 31%. One study used the Diagnostic and Statistical Manual of Mental Disorders of psychiatric illness (DSM III-R) and found 53% of patients exhibiting mental illness, 25% avoidance behavior, and 40% impaired well-being. The authors concluded that surgical treatment of penile cancer negatively effects well-being in up to 40% of patients with psychiatric symptoms in approximately 50%. Additionally, up to 75% of patients reported a reduction in sexual function after surgery.

Carcinoma In Situ (Tis) and Verrucous Carcinoma (Ta)

Penile squamous cell *carcinoma in situ*, also known as erythroplasia of Queyrat, is a well-marginated lesion of the glans or prepuce of uncircumcised men. After biopsy confirmation, a conservative approach that spares penile anatomy and function is preferred. Preputial lesions are adequately treated with circumcision. Topical 5-FU cream provides excellent cosmetic results for lesions of the glans and meatus. Long-term follow-up on patients treated with the combination of carbon dioxide and YAG lasers has shown good local tumor control and highly satisfactory cosmesis [5, 6]. Mohs micrographic surgery has

been described as a less deforming alternative to partial amputation though most require immediate tissue flap reconstruction [7]. Local control rates with a Mohs procedure range from 70 to 86% in selected patients [7, 8]. Radiation therapy may be used to eradicate these lesions with minimal morbidity and reported 100% local control rates for Tis [9].

Penile verrucous carcinoma is characterized by aggressive local growth and a low metastatic potential. Conservative therapeutic approaches are generally favored and partial or total penectomy may be considered overtreatment. Use of laser ablation, cryotherapy, or Mohs micrographic surgical technique has been described [10]. One study of intra-aortic infusion with methotrexate in four patients with verrucous carcinoma produced three complete remissions [11]. Although treatment with radiation is associated with concerns of malignant transformation, one series included nine such patients treated with radiation therapy and a reported 100% local control rate [12].

Invasive Cancer

As discussed above, surgical excision of penile cancer provides effective local control and remains the most common approach to penile carcinoma in the United States. However, because of the functional and psychosexual morbidity [4, 13] penile sparing treatment using radiation therapy with either brachytherapy or external beam radiation should be considered. Both techniques have been utilized since the 1950s [12] and demonstrate good local control with the advantage of preserving organ function in early-stage penile cancer [14–17]. Below we discuss techniques and outcomes of both modalities.

Brachytherapy

Patient Selection

Reported series of brachytherapy results for squamous carcinoma of the penis have not used strict selection criteria. Retrospective analysis can thus determine which features define the ideal patient with a high likelihood of treatment success and a low risk of complications. These criteria should not be used to exclude those patients who do not fulfill all features, but rather as a means of counseling patients as to their relative risk of an adverse outcome and to establish realistic expectations, thereby enabling them to decide amongst the various treatment options being presented.

Tumor Size

It is recognized that larger lesions require a greater volume implant with a higher number of needles portending a higher risk of both recurrence and complications such as soft tissue necrosis. The ideal tumor for brachytherapy should be less than 4 cm in maximal diameter. Kiltie et al. [18] described results for 31 patients treated over a 17-year period. Three of five patients (60%) with a tumor diameter >4 cm had a local failure as compared to 3 of 21 (14%) with a diameter <4 cm ($p=0.05$). Similarly, Mazeron et al. [19] treated very few tumors >4 cm but observed a local failure rate of 50% (2/4) for >4 cm as compared to 11% (2/19) for <2 cm and 26% (7/27) for 2–4 cm. However, a larger multi-institution French experience reported by Rozan et al. [14] among 184 patients reported a local failure rate of only 20% for tumors with a diameter >3 cm versus 14% if ≤3 cm ($p=0.05$). Although statistically significant, the difference was not sufficient to deny a patient with a larger tumor access to brachytherapy. De Crevoisier et al. [20] reported on 144 patients with Jackson Stage 1 penile cancers (median diameter 20 mm: range 2–50 mm) and found a tumor diameter >4 cm to predict for local recurrence but still reported a 10-year actuarial freedom from local failure of 50% among these patients. Crook et al. [21] also reported very good success with larger tumors in a series of 49 patients; although there were 19 tumors with a diameter >3 cm, size was not a predictive factor for local failure ($p=0.43$). This supports the philosophy that although local failure may be of greater risk with larger tumors, a strict size limit may not be appropriate.

Tumor Histology/Morphology

Squamous carcinoma is the most frequent pathology seen with insufficient reported experience on verrucous carcinoma or other subtypes. Results for brachytherapy have not been compared with respect to exophytic versus infiltrative morphology. However, when treating an apparently infiltrative tumor, care must be taken to have adequate depth of coverage, erring if necessary on the side of being overly generous. Rozan et al.'s [14] analysis of the French experience according to tumor morphology illustrates the problem with a reported local failure rate of 23% for infiltrative tumors versus 12% for non-infiltrative tumors ($p=0.05$). The depth of invasion is clearly evident for the experienced practitioner at the first post-implant follow-up visit 3–4 weeks after brachytherapy when tumor regression will have left a crater at the tumor site.

According to stage, Delannes et al. [22] reported local control in 91% of T1–T2 lesions versus 16.7% of T3 lesions. Rozan et al.'s [14] larger experience was not as dismal with local failures seen in 15% of T1, 16% of T2, and 23% of T3 tumors (6/26). This is similar to Mazeron et al. [19] where local failures were seen in 11% of T1 (1/9), 22% of T2 (6/27), and 29% of T3 (4/14) tumors.

Tumor Extent/Location

The most common sites for penile SCC are the glans and foreskin. Circumcision, in addition to providing full exposure of the lesion, will often remove a portion of it with the diseased foreskin. Brachytherapy is generally not recommended for tumors originating on the shaft of the penis or at the base. Although these sites may be technically amenable to implantation, published experience is currently lacking. Brachytherapy of a lesion on the shaft is likely to impair erections, and may result in subsequent curvature.

A more common scenario is when a lesion straddles the coronal sulcus, involving the glans, foreskin, and portion of the shaft. Provided the overall dimensions are not excessive, such lesions can be treated with brachytherapy especially if the extension on the shaft is minimal and can be encompassed with one additional treatment plane.

Tumor Grade

Few series have analyzed outcome stratified by grade. Crook et al. [23] found grade to be a significant determinant of disease-free survival ($p=0.003$), with 39% of patients with moderately or poorly differentiated tumors experiencing regional or distant failure but with no influence on local control. Grade should clearly be a determinant of groin management but does not preclude brachytherapy in the management of the primary tumor.

Technique

Since squamous carcinoma of the penis most frequently occurs in the uncircumcised and often under a phimotic or nonretractile foreskin, full exposure of the lesion through circumcision is essential. This should be performed prior to the procedure; 10–14 days are generally sufficient for healing. Brachytherapy can be performed under general, spinal, or local anesthesia. The procedure generally takes under an hour and begins with insertion of a Foley catheter and then careful identification of the extent of tumor through inspection and palpation. Imaging of the primary tumor to determine the depth of invasion is not routinely done although ultrasound or MRI with artificially induced erection have been reported [24], and may be helpful in the planning process. The extent of disease and planned dosing coverage should be drawn using a sterile marker pen, aiming for the prescription isodose to fall at least 1 cm beyond visible or palpable disease.

The next step in the implant procedure is to plan the placement of the source-carrier needles. Penile brachytherapy involves through-and-through insertion of multiple parallel planes of needles. The depth of invasion of the tumor is frequently underappreciated and for this reason, single-plane implants and surface

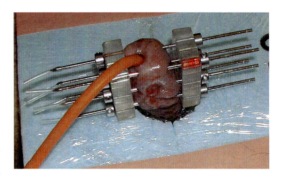

Fig. 8.1 Pulse dose rate brachytherapy implant showing a 2-plane, 6-needle implant with urinary catheter in place and protective styrofoam support to distance the implanted site from the neighboring structures

applicators are discouraged as they may result in underdosing of the tumor at a depth. To maintain parallelism, some form of fixation is required. Predrilled transparent Lucite or plexiglass templates are ideal and can be positioned on either side of the penis, and fixed in place for the duration of the implant (Fig. 8.1) [25]. Many smaller tumors can be treated within two planes but more deeply invasive or larger tumors will require three or sometimes four planes of treatment. Ideal spacing between the needles and planes for low-dose-rate (LDR) brachytherapy is 15–18 mm. When all the needles have been satisfactorily positioned, each one must be locked in position using either metal buttons which can be crimped around the needle against the outside surface of each template or preferably a locking collar fixed with a tiny screw which is tightened perpendicular to the needle. Precise measurements are taken of the protrusion lengths of each needle beyond the template and the spacing between the templates. A geometrically stable structure has been created which will maintain its shape and position for the duration of the treatment. A styrofoam or sponge collar can be fashioned around the base of the penis for support and to distance the distal implant site from neighboring structures.

For LDR brachytherapy, the prescribed dose is usually 60 Gy, delivered at a dose rate of 50–60 cGy/h. The duration of the implant is thus 100–120 h (i.e., 4–5 days). Much of the reported experience has depended on the Paris System of dosimetry for guidance in dose prescription

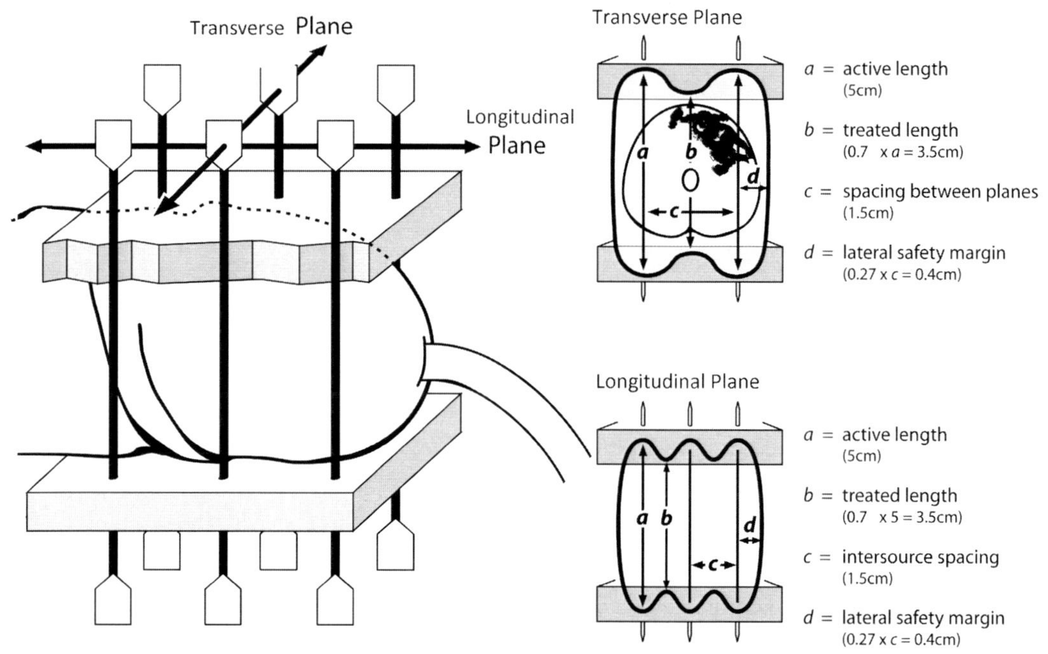

Transverse Plane

Longitudinal Plane

Transverse Plane

a = active length (5cm)

b = treated length (0.7 x a = 3.5cm)

c = spacing between planes (1.5cm)

d = lateral safety margin (0.27 x c = 0.4cm)

Longitudinal Plane

a = active length (5cm)

b = treated length (0.7 x 5 = 3.5cm)

c = intersource spacing (1.5cm)

d = lateral safety margin (0.27 x c = 0.4cm)

Fig. 8.2 Diagram of an idealized "Paris system" implant very similar to the clinical photo illustration in Fig. 8.1. The mathematical relationship between the location of the prescription isodose and the spacing and length of the needles is shown (adapted from Crook J, Jezioranski J, Cygler JE. Penile brachytherapy: technical aspects and postimplant issues. Brachytherapy 2010 Apr-Jun;9(2): 151–158)

[14, 18–20, 22, 23]. Dose rate minima are calculated in a plane perpendicular to the needles (basal dose rate) and then the dose prescribed at the isodose representing 85% of this dose rate (reference isodose). Simple mathematical relationships have been described to estimate at the time of implantation where the prescription isodose will fall relative to the needles based on the spacing between them and the treated distance between the two templates (Fig. 8.2). Treatment can be delivered using either continuous LDR or automated afterloading pulse dose rate (PDR) brachytherapy. The patient remains hospitalized for the duration of the treatment but once the needles are positioned and stabilized, discomfort is usually minimal. In the past, most LDR implants were performed with manually after-loaded iridium-192 radioactive wires loaded into the carrier needles after they were positioned and fixed in place. In the present day, the same radiobiologic effect can be achieved using automated afterloading with a PDR machine at the bedside, programmed to deliver one pulse per hour [26]. A single radioactive bead steps through each of

the source-carrier needles in turn, delivering the same 50–60 cGy in an hourly pulse that would have been delivered each hour by the continuously emitting wires. Each pulse takes 5–10 min. The use of PDR delivery eliminates radiation exposure to the brachytherapist at the time of the procedure, as well as to other healthcare workers and nurses involved in patient care.

High-dose-rate (HDR) brachytherapy is gradually replacing LDR in many tumor sites and HDR afterloaders are widely available in most radiotherapy departments. However, there is as yet very little published experience on HDR brachytherapy for penile cancer. HDR implants require closer needle spacing to maintain a greater degree of homogeneity. The ideal spacing is 9–12 mm, and can be variable within the same implant since the dose distribution can be optimized by varying the dwell times as the source steps through the carrier needles. Petera et al. [27] reported on ten patients treated with HDR using a fractionation of 3 Gy twice daily for 9 days. This somewhat prolonged fractionation for a brachytherapy procedure can probably be safely reduced to 3.2–3.4 Gy given twice daily over 6 days provided careful attention is paid to the homogeneity of the dose distribution. To reduce the risk of late complications, the volume of tissue receiving 150% of the prescribed dose should be limited to 20% of the implanted volume and the volume receiving 125% limited to 40%. Otherwise, the implant procedure is quite similar to the LDR technique.

Results

A summary of the pertinent literature is shown in Table 8.1. The majority of tumors treated are T1–T2 (invasion into corpus spongiosum or cavernosum but not involving the urethra) or Jackson Stage 1 (limited to glans and prepuce with no involvement of the shaft) although many series have a small number of treated T3 or Jackson stage 2 tumors. Successful control of the primary tumor with brachytherapy at 5 years is 75–87%, and at 10 years 72–80%. Several series report late recurrences beyond 5 years and for this reason extended follow-up is recommended for 10 years and beyond [19, 20, 23]. As late failures are successfully salvaged with surgery, cause-specific survival does not drop between 5 and 10 years in many series, with reported rates of 84–92%. Ultimate penile preservation rates at 10 years of 67–70% have been reported.

Complications

The most common late side effects are soft tissue necrosis at the implant site (0–23%), and meatal stenosis (9–45%). Expected late sequelae albeit minor include mild dyschromia and telangiectasia. Although not consistently reported, brachytherapy at a distal location on the penis does not appear to impair erectile function.

Soft tissue necrosis or late ulceration increases in frequency with implant volume, tumor size, tumor stage, and dose. De Crevoisier et al. [20] reported a 10-year actuarial rate of 26% painful soft tissue ulceration at a prescribed dose of 65 Gy, while Crook et al. [23] reported a rate of

12% for a prescribed dose of 60 Gy. De Crevoisier et al. [20] performed a multivariate analysis for predictors of ulceration and found implant volume (RR 1.02, 95% CI 1.01–1.03) and dose rate (RR 9.17, 95% CI 1.8–46.6) to be predictive. Both Crook et al. and De Crevoisier et al. [20] used Paris system guidelines for implant geometry and dose prescription but the more tightly controlled dose rate achievable with PDR brachytherapy in Crook's series [23] may account for the much lower complication rate. Rozan et al. [14] similarly reported higher complication rates in patients with implants >30 cc, more than two planes of implant needles, and total prescribed dose >60 Gy. Mazeron et al. [19] reported increased painful ulceration for T3 tumors, occurring in two of five patients, and also found healing to be delayed beyond 3 months in larger volume implants. Soft tissue ulceration can be successfully managed conservatively with attention to hygiene, antibiotics, and vitamin E ointment. If conservative measures fail, hyperbaric oxygen will often promote healing and avoid the need for amputation [28].

Meatal stenosis can often be managed conservatively by self-dilatation with a meatal dilator as required. As this is more successful if initiated early at the first signs of a narrow or deviated urinary stream, some centers of excellence routinely supply patients with a meatal dilator at the first post-implant visit. De Crevoisier et al. [20] reported a 10-year actuarial meatal stenosis rate of 29% but defined this as requiring any use of meatal self-dilatation. None of their cases required surgical intervention, whereas three of eight patients with meatal stenosis in Mazeron et al.'s [19] series did undergo surgical urethral reconstruction.

Summary of Brachytherapy

Brachytherapy for penile cancer is an effective penile conserving option. The ideal patient would have a T1–T2 tumor <4 cm in maximum diameter, without extensive infiltration of the corpora cavernosa or extension beyond the coronal sulcus. Grade does not appear to influence local

Table 8.1 Summary of results for interstitial brachytherapy for penile cancer

Author/year	Years spanned	n	Stage	Dose Gray (range)	f/up (years)	LC by RT	CSS	Penile preservation	Necrosis	Meatal stenosis	Notes
Chaudhary, 1999 [39]	1988–96	23	T1: 7, T2: 7 Rec: 9	50 (40–60)	2 (0.3–9.8)	18/23 70% at 8 years	ns	70% at 8 years		2/23	
Crook, 2009 [23]	1989–2007	67	T1: 56%, T2: 33% T3: 8%, 38% >3 cm	60	4 (0.5–16)	87% at 5 years 72% at 10 years	83.6% at 5 and 10 year	88% at 5 years 67% at 10 years	12%		No effect of size (to 5 cm) or grade on LF
De Crevoisier, 2009 [20]	1970–2006	144	100% Jackson 1 Med diam 20 mm 81% sup/19% inf/ulc	65 (37–75)	5.7 (0.5–29)	80% at 10 years	92% at 10 years	70% at 10 years	26%	29%	Not BT if extends beyond glans ↓dose rate if large
Delannes, 1992 [22]	1971–89	51	T1: 14, T2: 28 T3: 6	60 (50–65)	5.5 [1–12]	44/51 crude 86% at 5 years	85% at 5 and 10 years	67% 71% T1–2	23%	45%	↑LF if ↑ size >4 cm or volume
Kiltie, 2000 [18]	1980–97	31	Jackson1: 27 Jackson2: 4	63.5 (60–66.5)	5.1 (0.3–14)	25/31 81%	85.4% 5 years	75% 5 years	8%	44%	↑LF if ↑ size >4 cm, T2 or ↑volume
Mazeron, 1984 [19]	1970–79	50	T1: 9,T2: 27 T3: 14	65 (60–70)	3–8+	78% crude		74%	6%	16%	↑LF if size >4 cm, or deep infiltration
Rozan, 1995 [14]	1959–89	184	Jackson1:93% Jackson2: 7%	63 (10–87)	11.6 (2.5–32)	86%	88% at 5 and 10 years	78%	21%	45%	
Soria, 1996 [12]	1973–93	72	T1: 67, T2: 24 T3: 6	61–70	9.3 (2.5–32)	77%	72% at 5 years 62% at 10 years	75% at 5 years 68% at 10 years	ns	ns	Probable overlap with De Crevoisier
Petera, 2011 [27]	2002–09	10	T1–T2	HDR BT 54/18/9d	2	100%	100%	100%	0	0	

Rec: recurrent
Sup/inf/ulc: superficial/infiltrative/ulcerated
LC: local control
LF: local failure

control rates. Moderate increase in the risk of local recurrence or complications such as soft tissue ulceration are seen with T3 tumors or larger volume implants but this does not preclude brachytherapy being considered as an option under such circumstances provided the patient and referring physicians are aware. Close follow-up and prompt salvage surgical resection if required will prevent local recurrences from impacting the likelihood of a favorable disease-specific survival.

External Beam Radiation Therapy

EBRT has been used successfully in the definitive management of invasive carcinoma of the penis for over 6 decades. However, due to the rarity of penile cancer, outcome data is often limited to single-center retrospective series. Definitive EBRT is most appropriate for T1, T2, and selected T3 tumors [14]. Treatment of tumors >4 cm with EBRT alone is discouraged since local failure rates approach 75% [29, 30]. T3 and T4 lesions may be treated with radiation in a neoadjuvant fashion prior to surgery, with or without concurrent chemotherapy, or in selected postoperative cases [31].

Outcomes with EBRT

Local control rates for T1–2 penile cancer treated with EBRT range from 65 to 81%, with one report of a 90% local control rate in a small series of only ten patients [32]. Table 8.2 provides a summary of treatment outcomes for EBRT, with organ preservation rates ranging from 39 to 85%. Most local failures can be salvaged with surgery consisting of either local excision or more frequently, partial or total penectomy. Given the success of salvage surgery for radiation failures, it is reasonable to treat primarily with radiation therapy reserving surgery for local failures. Equivalent overall survival has been reported for this approach compared to primary surgery [33].

Most published results span several decades during which time radiation therapy techniques

would be considered inadequate by modern standards. Often the prescribed dose was suboptimal for squamous cell carcinoma. Sarin et al. have reported inferior local control with doses <60 Gy ($p = 0.11$), fraction sizes <2 Gy, and treatment duration >45 days [31]. Zouhair et al. found that 9 of 14 local failures received doses <64 Gy [33]. Based on the experience obtained from the care of other squamous cell cancers, doses of 66–70 Gy are required to optimize local control. Rozan et al. found a local control rate approaching 90% in 20 patients treated with dose escalation using EBRT followed by a brachytherapy boost [14].

Postoperative Radiation

Radiation therapy may be employed after surgical intervention of the primary tumor [12, 34] but the indications for postoperative radiation and its impact on local control or survival are unclear. One Austrian study reported on postoperative radiation for positive margins at the primary site in 24 patients [31], 7 after total penectomy, 10 after partial penectomy, and 7 after local excision. Radiation consisted of 50–60 Gy of EBRT or 45 Gy of brachytherapy. Five-year local control, progression-free, and overall survival rates were 75, 87, and 57%, respectively.

Lymph Node Irradiation

For patients with T1 or T2, N0 cancers that are Grade 1–2, prophylactic lymph node irradiation is not necessary [29, 30]. For Grade 3 or more advanced disease, elective nodal irradiation should be considered if staging ILND is not performed. For node-positive patients, irradiation of the involved regional lymph nodes may cure some patients and is an alternative when surgical excision is not possible. In one series [35], 13 patients with involved regional lymph nodes received radiation therapy with 38% of patients surviving at 5 years. Ozsahin et al. reported on 18 patients with lymph node involvement [34] of whom 11 underwent inguinal lymphadenectomy

Table 8.2 Summary of results for EBRT for penile cancer

Author	Number of patients	Treatment	Total dose (Gy)	5 year LC %	Salvage surgery, N	Late complications
Rozan [14]	75	EBRT+BT	59+40.5	88%	27	5 penis necrosis
McLean [9]	26	EBRT	35–60	61%	5	7 urethral stenosis or phimosis
Modig [33]	25	EBRT+bleomycin	56–58	75%	5	1 urethral stenosis
Sarin [30]	75	EBRT±BT	70	66	26	7 urethral stenosis and/or stricture
Neave [37]	20	EBRT	50–55	n/a	n/a	2 urethral strictures
Soria [12]	72	BT±EBRT	60–70		18	
Zouhair [36]	23	EBRT±BT	45–74	41	14	2 urethral stenosis
Azrif [29]	41	EBRT	50–52.5	62%	n/a	3 penile ulceration, 11 urethral stenosis
Sagerman [40]	24	EBRT	45–64	75% at 3 years	n/a	n/a
Kaushal [41]	16	EBRT	55	81%	3	2 meatal stenosis

and postoperative radiation therapy while the other 7 received radiation alone. There were four regional failures, two in the postoperative group and two in the EBRT-alone group. Similar results were reported by Zouhair et al. who treated 12 patients with clinically positive lymph nodes; 5 underwent inguinal lymphadenectomy plus postoperative radiation while 7 had radiation alone [36]. There were three regional failures, two with surgery and one with radiation. Results are less favorable among those with more advanced disease. In a series from the Royal Marsden Hospital, regional control was accomplished in only two of six patients with N1, two of five with N2, and one of seven patients with N3 disease [30].

Side Effects of Treatment

Acute reactions such as swelling, discomfort, and desquamation are usually self-limited. Care should be taken to avoid secondary infections that may result from skin breakdown. The use of large fraction sizes should be avoided to reduce the risk of late radiation effects such as fibrosis. The incidence of urethral strictures and/or stenosis has been reported to be between 4 and 49% [9, 30, 33, 36, 37]. Penile necrosis may as well occur but is more often associated with brachytherapy [14]. The majority of patients (up to 90%) are able to maintain erectile function following radiation therapy [32, 38].

EBRT Technique

When delivering external-beam megavoltage, radiation beams (4–6 MV) are typically employed with a tissue-equivalent bolus (usually wax or plastic) to provide sufficient dose buildup on the surface of the lesion. All patients should first undergo circumcision if they have not already done so. The penis is then suspended and surrounded by bolus above the pelvis. Though the entire penile shaft has been traditionally treated, it is now recommended that for T1–2, N0 cancers <4 cm, only the tumor plus a 2 cm margin be targeted. Additionally, it is not recommended that either the groin or pelvic nodes be treated in such low-risk patients [29]. For T3–4 or >4 cm tumors or node-positive patients, pelvic and inguinal lymph node irradiation is recommended with or without concomitant chemotherapy. When treating the pelvic nodes, the penis can be secured cranially into the pelvic field and hence irradiated.

For T1–2, <4 cm, N0 tumors typical doses are 65–70 Gy to the gross tumor volume (GTV) + 2 cm margin in a standard fractionation (1.8–2 Gy/day). Hypofractionation should be avoided. For T3–4, >4 cm, or N1–3 disease the pelvis, inguinal, and whole penile shaft should be treated initially to a dose of 45–50.4 Gy, and perform a boost to the GTV plus 2 cm margin for a total dose of 64–70 Gy.

In the postoperative setting among patients with positive inguinal lymph nodes, one should treat the inguinal and pelvic lymph nodes to a dose of 45–50.4 Gy with a boosting of gross nodes or regions of extracapsular extension to doses of 60–66 Gy. Concomitant chemotherapy should be considered, though there is no evidence base for such an approach in penile cancer but rather is an extrapolation from scientific literature pertaining to other disease sites. Treatment of the primary site of disease should be included for positive margins and considered in cases of close or indeterminant surgical margins. In instances where there is a positive surgical margin, treatment should be directed to the primary site of disease and the surgical scar to doses of 60–66 Gy.

Conclusion

Squamous carcinoma of the penis is an uncommon tumor in developed nations. Recent guidelines from both the European and American Urologic Associations favor a penile sparing approach whenever possible. Radiation therapy in the form of either brachytherapy or EBRT provides comparable survival rates with the added benefit of preserving an often functionally intact phallus and therefore should be considered at centers of excellence where this expertise is available.

References

1. Brkovic D, Kalble T, Dorsam J, Pomer S, Lotzerich C, Banafsche R, et al. Surgical treatment of invasive penile cancer—the Heidelberg experience from 1968 to 1994. Eur Urol. 1997;31(3):339–42.
2. Horenblas S, van Tinteren H, Delemarre JF, Boon TA, Moonen LM, Lustig V. Squamous cell carcinoma of the penis. II. Treatment of the primary tumor. J Urol. 1992;147(6):1533–8.
3. Opjordsmoen S, Waehre H, Aass N, Fossa SD. Sexuality in patients treated for penile cancer: patients' experience and doctors' judgement. Br J Urol. 1994; 73(5):554–60.
4. Maddineni SB, Lau MM, Sangar VK. Identifying the needs of penile cancer sufferers: a systematic review of the quality of life, psychosexual and psychosocial literature in penile cancer. BMC Urol. 2009;9:8.
5. Windahl T, Andersson SO. Combined laser treatment for penile carcinoma: results after long-term followup. J Urol. 2003;169(6):2118–21.
6. Frimberger D, Hungerhuber E, Zaak D, Waidelich R, Hofstetter A, Schneede P. Penile carcinoma. Is Nd:YAG laser therapy radical enough? J Urol. 2002; 168(6):2418–21. Discussion 2421.
7. Shindel AW, Mann MW, Lev RY, Sengelmann R, Petersen J, Hruza GJ, et al. Mohs micrographic surgery for penile cancer: management and long-term followup. J Urol. 2007;178(5):1980–5.
8. Mohs FE, Snow SN, Larson PO. Mohs micrographic surgery for penile tumors. Urol Clin North Am. 1992; 19(2):291–304.
9. McLean M, Akl AM, Warde P, Bissett R, Panzarella T, Gospodarowicz M. The results of primary radiation therapy in the management of squamous cell carcinoma of the penis. Int J Radiat Oncol Biol Phys. 1993;25(4):623–8.
10. Michelman FA, Filho AC, Moraes AM. Verrucous carcinoma of the penis treated with cryosurgery. J Urol. 2002;168(3):1096–7.
11. Sheen MC, Sheu HM, Huang CH, Wang YW, Chai CY, Wu CF. Penile verrucous carcinoma successfully treated by intra-aortic infusion with methotrexate. Urology. 2003;61(6):1216–20.
12. Soria JC, Fizazi K, Piron D, Kramar A, Gerbaulet A, Haie-Meder C, et al. Squamous cell carcinoma of the penis: multivariate analysis of prognostic factors and natural history in monocentric study with a conservative policy. Ann Oncol. 1997;8(11):1089–98.
13. Hanash KA, Furlow WL, Utz DC, Harrison Jr EG. Carcinoma of the penis: a clinicopathologic study. J Urol. 1970;104(2):291–7.
14. Rozan R, Albuisson E, Giraud B, Donnarieix D, Delannes M, Pigneux J, et al. Interstitial brachytherapy for penile carcinoma: a multicentric survey (259 patients). Radiother Oncol. 1995;36(2):83–93.
15. Gerbaulet A, Lambin P. Radiation therapy of cancer of the penis. Indications, advantages, and pitfalls. Urol Clin North Am. 1992;19(2):325–32.
16. Haile K, Delclos L. The place of radiation therapy in the treatment of carcinoma of the distal end of the penis. Cancer. 1980;45(7 Suppl):1980–4.
17. Ardiet JM, Gerard JP, Romestaing P, de Laroche G, Montarbon JF, Chassard JL, et al. Treatment, by 192-iridium curietherapy, of epitheliomas of the penis. Apropos of 36 cases. J Urol. 1984;90(8–9):557–61.
18. Kiltie AE, Elwell C, Close HJ, Ash DV. Iridium-192 implantation for node-negative carcinoma of the penis: the Cookridge Hospital experience. Clin Oncol (R Coll Radiol). 2000;12(1):25–31.
19. Mazeron JJ, Langlois D, Lobo PA, Huart JA, Calitchi E, Lusinchi A, et al. Interstitial radiation therapy for carcinoma of the penis using iridium 192 wires: the Henri Mondor experience (1970–1979). Int J Radiat Oncol Biol Phys. 1984;10(10):1891–5.
20. de Crevoisier R, Slimane K, Sanfilippo N, Bossi A, Albano M, Dumas I, et al. Long-term results of brachytherapy for carcinoma of the penis confined to the glans (N- or NX). Int J Radiat Oncol Biol Phys. 2009;74(4):1150–6.
21. Crook J, Grimard L, Tsihlias J, Morash C, Panzarella T. Interstitial brachytherapy for penile cancer: an alternative to amputation. J Urol. 2002;167(2 Pt 1):506–11.
22. Delannes M, Malavaud B, Douchez J, Bonnet J, Daly NJ. Iridium-192 interstitial therapy for squamous cell carcinoma of the penis. Int J Radiat Oncol Biol Phys. 1992;24(3):479–83.
23. Crook J, Ma C, Grimard L. Radiation therapy in the management of the primary penile tumor: an update. World J Urol. 2009;27(2):189.
24. Lont AP, Besnard AP, Gallee MP, van Tinteren H, Horenblas S. A comparison of physical examination and imaging in determining the extent of primary penile carcinoma. BJU Int. 2003;91(6):493–5.
25. Crook J, Jezioranski J, Cygler JE. Penile brachytherapy: technical aspects and post implant issues. Brachytherapy. 2010;9(2):151–8.
26. Dale RG, Jones B. The clinical radiobiology of brachytherapy. Br J Radiol. 1998;71(845):465–83.
27. Petera J, Sirak I, Kasaova L, Macingova Z, Paluska P, Zouhar M, et al. High-dose rate brachytherapy in the treatment of penile carcinoma—first experience. Brachytherapy. 2011;10(2):136–40.
28. Gomez-Iturriaga A, Crook J, Evans W, Saibishkumar EP, Jezioranski J. The efficacy of hyperbaric oxygen therapy in the treatment of medically refractory soft tissue necrosis after penile brachytherapy. Brachytherapy. 2011;10(6):491–7.
29. Azrif M, Logue JP, Swindell R, Cowan RA, Wylie JP, Livsey JE. External-beam radiotherapy in T1-2 N0 penile carcinoma. Clin Oncol (R Coll Radiol). 2006;18(4):320–5.
30. Sarin R, Norman AR, Steel GG, Horwich A. Treatment results and prognostic factors in 101 men treated for squamous carcinoma of the penis. Int J Radiat Oncol Biol Phys. 1997;38(4):713–22.
31. Langsenlehner T, Mayer R, Quehenberger F, Prettenhofer U, Langsenlehner U, Pummer K, et al.

The role of radiation therapy after incomplete resection of penile cancer. Strahlenther Onkol. 2008;184(7):359–63.

32. Grabstald H, Kelley CD. Radiation therapy of penile cancer: six to ten-year follow-up. Urology. 1980;15(6):575–6.

33. Modig H, Duchek M, Sjodin JG. Carcinoma of the penis. Treatment by surgery or combined bleomycin and radiation therapy. Acta Oncol. 1993;32(6):653–5.

34. Ozsahin M, Jichlinski P, Weber DC, Azria D, Zimmermann M, Guillou L, et al. Treatment of penile carcinoma: to cut or not to cut? Int J Radiat Oncol Biol Phys. 2006;66(3):674–9.

35. Staubitz WJ, Lent MH, Oberkircher OJ. Carcinoma of the penis. Cancer. 1955;8(2):371–8.

36. Zouhair A, Coucke PA, Jeanneret W, Douglas P, Do HP, Jichlinski P, et al. Radiation therapy alone or combined surgery and radiation therapy in squamous-cell carcinoma of the penis? Eur J Cancer. 2001;37(2):198–203.

37. Neave F, Neal AJ, Hoskin PJ, Hope-Stone HF. Carcinoma of the penis: a retrospective review of treatment with iridium mould and external beam irradiation. Clin Oncol (R Coll Radiol). 1993;5(4):207–10.

38. Krieg RM, Luk KH. Carcinoma of penis. Review of cases treated by surgery and radiation therapy 1960–1977. Urology. 1981;18(2):149–54.

39. Chaudhary AJ, Ghosh S, Bhalavat RL, Kulkarni JN, Sequeira BV. Interstitial brachytherapy in carcinoma of the penis. Strahlenther Onkol. 1999;175(1):17–20.

40. Sagerman RH, Yu WS, Chung CT, Puranik A, Duncan W, Jackson SM. External-beam irradiation of carcinoma of the penis. The treatment of early cancer of the penis with megavoltage X-rays. Radiology. 1984;152(1):183–5.

41. Kaushal V, Sharma SC. Carcinoma of the penis. A 12-year review. Acta Oncol. 1987;26(6):413–7.

Multimodal Approach to the Management of Locally Advanced and Metastatic Penile Cancer

9

Lance C. Pagliaro and Curtis A. Pettaway

Abbreviations

5-FU   5-Fluorouracil
BMP   Bleomycin, methotrexate, and cisplatin
EGFR   Epidermal growth factor receptor
EORTC   European Organization for Research and Treatment of Cancer
HPV   Human papillomavirus
MMC   Mitomycin-C
PF   Cisplatin plus 5-FU

Introduction

The role of combined-modality therapy in the treatment of penile cancer has been becoming better defined [1, 2]. Surgery and radiotherapy have long been the mainstay of therapy for penile cancer [3–6]. A multidisciplinary treatment approach has been elusive, however, because patients are more commonly treated with surgery or radiation alone, or with both done sequentially. Postoperative radiotherapy to the inguinal regions and soft tissues of the

pelvis carries specific risks, including skin breakdown, impaired wound healing, and chronic lower-extremity edema. There have been no randomized clinical trials, so data are lacking on the relative merits of lymphadenectomy alone, in the case of regional lymph node metastases, versus radiotherapy or a multimodal approach.

The development of multimodal therapy for locally advanced and metastatic penile cancer has also been hampered by the lack of systemic therapy options with proven efficacy. For some disease sites, systemic chemotherapy has been successfully combined with radiotherapy, such as mitomycin-C (MMC) and 5-fluorouracil (5-FU) for anal cancer [7], and docetaxel, 5-FU, and cisplatin for squamous cell carcinoma of the head and neck [8]. In other disease sites, such as the colon, breast, and bladder, adjuvant or neoadjuvant chemotherapy has resulted in improved surgical outcomes. This chapter discusses the role of systemic therapy in penile cancer and its integration with surgery or radiotherapy in the contemporary standard of care.

Dissemination of penile cancer occurs through the lymphatics, first to the inguinal lymph nodes and then to the pelvic nodes. Only about 2% of patients present initially with distant metastases. The far more common presentation is metastatic disease confined to regional lymph nodes. Patients with high-risk features in the primary tumor and clinically negative groins have about a 40% risk of harboring occult lymph node metastases. Tumor involvement of the inguinal lymph nodes

L.C. Pagliaro, M.D. (✉)
Department of Genitourinary Medical Oncology,
The University of Texas MD Anderson Cancer Center,
1515 Holcombe Blvd., Houston, TX 77030, USA
e-mail: lpagliar@mdanderson.org

C.A. Pettaway, M.D.
Department of Urology, University of Texas MD
Anderson Cancer Center, Houston, TX, USA

is associated with increased risk of death from penile cancer. The prognosis varies, depending on the extent of lymph node involvement. The subset of patients with "bulky" inguinal lymph nodes (i.e., greater than 4 cm, fixed, ulcerated, or found to have extranodal extension) are rarely cured with surgery alone [1, 9, 10]. Metastases to pelvic lymph nodes also have an 80–90% risk of recurrence and death after pelvic lymphadenectomy alone. These are patients for whom a multimodality approach is clearly desirable, with the goal of improving survival.

Retrospective Data

Historically, chemotherapy for penile cancer was fraught with unacceptable toxicity, low response rates, and a median overall survival duration of only about 7 months [11]. The largest phase II clinical trial of chemotherapy for metastatic penile cancer to date was the Southwest Oncology Group study of bleomycin, methotrexate, and cisplatin (BMP); the overall response rate was 32.5%, and several patients died from pulmonary toxicity associated with bleomycin. Cisplatin plus 5-FU (PF) was subsequently used as a standard regimen in Europe, although there has not yet been a large prospective study of this combination in penile cancer [12, 13]. In 2007, Leitje et al. [14] reported on a retrospective series of 20 patients with regional lymph node metastases who had been given BMP, PF, or other chemotherapy prior to planned surgical resection. Patients whose tumors responded to that neoadjuvant chemotherapy regimen had a much better overall survival duration than did those whose tumors did not respond (Fig. 9.1).

In a retrospective series from The University of Texas MD Anderson Cancer Center, ten patients were described who had undergone inguinal and pelvic lymph node dissections after having experienced an objective response or stable disease while receiving neoadjuvant chemotherapy [15]. The regimens included BMP and combinations with paclitaxel. Three patients, all of whom had received a paclitaxel-containing regimen, had pathologic complete responses. Investigators in Europe have also reported encouraging preliminary results with taxanes in the neoadjuvant setting [16]. There still has been no randomized clinical trial, however, because penile cancer is a rare disease, making it difficult to conduct a large randomized study. Nevertheless, the gathering evidence suggested that survival of patients with locally advanced or metastatic penile cancer might be improved with neoadjuvant chemotherapy followed by inguinal and pelvic lymph node dissections.

There has also been interest in using chemotherapy for radiosensitization, i.e., concurrent chemoradiotherapy, for locoregionally metastatic

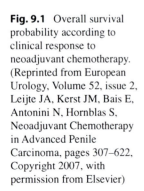

Fig. 9.1 Overall survival probability according to clinical response to neoadjuvant chemotherapy. (Reprinted from European Urology, Volume 52, issue 2, Leijte JA, Kerst JM, Bais E, Antonini N, Hornblas S, Neoadjuvant Chemotherapy in Advanced Penile Carcinoma, pages 307–622, Copyright 2007, with permission from Elsevier)

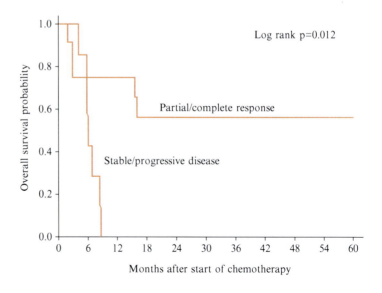

penile cancer [2]. There have not been any clinical trials specifically focused on chemoradiotherapy for penile cancer, but it has been used successfully in the treatment of squamous cell carcinoma at other disease sites. Examples of radiosensitizing chemotherapy include weekly cisplatin for cervical cancer [17], 5-FU and MMC for anal cancer [7], and PF for vulvar cancer [18, 19].

With respect to radiotherapy for metastatic penile cancer, administration of cisplatin alone or concurrently with 5-FU, or 5-FU and MMC, may result in better local tumor control than that provided by radiotherapy alone, especially for bulky tumors. However, the risks of toxicity and systemic failure associated with chemoradiation in this disease are uncertain and require further study. The optimal chemosensitizing regimen has not yet been defined, and overall and progression-free survival with chemoradiotherapy compared with surgery (alone or with neoadjuvant chemotherapy) have not yet been studied.

Prospective Study of Neoadjuvant Chemotherapy

A phase II study of combination therapy with irinotecan and cisplatin was performed by the European Organization for Research and Treatment of Cancer (EORTC) and reported in 2008 [20]. The authors described a neoadjuvant subgroup of seven patients who had stage T3 and/or N1 and/or N2 disease at baseline and who received a median of four cycles of chemotherapy. There were two objective responses (one complete, one partial), for an overall response rate of 28.6%. Three of the seven patients had undergone a lymphadenectomy following chemotherapy and were found to have no viable tumor remaining. This evidence was proof of principle that cisplatin-based chemotherapy in the neoadjuvant setting could yield meaningful responses and adds to the retrospective data, but there were too few patients to lead to definitive conclusions. Furthermore, the response rate for irinotecan and cisplatin in the entire study ($n = 26$) was 30.8%, no better than the historical rate with BMP [11].

Table 9.1 A neoadjuvant chemotherapy regimen (TIP)

Agent	Dose (mg/m^2)	Schedule	Notes
Paclitaxel	175	Day 1 over 3 h	Corticosteroid and antihistamines are given for hypersensitivity prophylaxis
Ifosfamide	1,200	Days 1–3	Mesna is given for urothelial protection
Cisplatin	25	Days 1–3	Mannitol is given with hydration after cisplatin

The cycle is repeated every 21 days, usually with granulocyte colony-stimulating factor prophylaxis beginning in the second cycle

A phase II study of neoadjuvant chemotherapy for patients with Tx N2–3 M0 disease was conducted at MD Anderson and reported in 2010 [21]. This 30-patient study was the first dedicated prospective study of a multimodal treatment in penile cancer. Patients were given four courses of paclitaxel, ifosfamide, and cisplatin (Table 9.1) before undergoing planned bilateral inguinal lymph node dissection and unilateral or bilateral pelvic lymph node dissection. All 30 patients received at least one course of chemotherapy, and 23 of them (76.7%) completed all four planned courses. The overall response rate was 50%, and 22 of the patients underwent surgery. Three patients (10%) were found to have no viable tumor remaining. At a median follow-up time of 34 months, nine patients (30%) were alive and disease free; two patients had died of other causes without experiencing recurrence. In a univariate analysis, time to disease progression and overall survival time were both significantly better in the patients whose tumors had responded to chemotherapy (Fig. 9.2) and whose post-chemotherapy residual lymph node disease was neither bilateral nor had extracapsular extension (Table 9.2). Postsurgical complications were comparable to or lower than those expected on the basis of contemporary series.

The MD Anderson study was not a randomized trial and was not designed to compare outcomes of neoadjuvant chemotherapy versus surgery alone. It is necessary, however, to consider the results in relation to historical experience because a randomized trial would not be feasible in such a rare

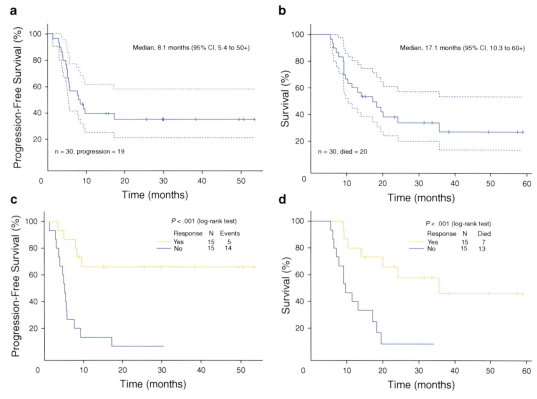

Fig. 9.2 Kaplan-Meier plots (with 95% confidence intervals as *dotted lines*) of (**a**) time to progression of disease and (**b**) overall survival; patients are grouped by response for (**c**) time to progression and (**d**) overall survival. Treatment consisted of neoadjuvant paclitaxel, ifosfamide, and cisplatin. (Pagliaro LC, Williams DL, Daliani D, Williams MB, Osai W, Kincaid M, et al., Neoadjuvant paclitaxel, ifosfamide, and cisplatin chemotherapy for metastatic penile cancer: A phase II study. J Clin Oncol 28, 2010:3851–3857. Reprinted with permission. © 2010 American Society of Clinical Oncology. All rights reserved)

Table 9.2 Histopathologic data on residual tumor from the 22 patients who completed all four courses of neoadjuvant chemotherapy and then underwent lymphadenectomy

Presence of histopathologic finding	Number (%) of patients	Univariate analyses			
		Median TTP (months)	Log-rank P value	Median OS (months)	Log-rank P value
Bilateral residual metastatic tumor					
Yes	8 (36.4)	5		10	
No	14 (63.6)[a]	>50	0.002	36	0.017
Extranodal extension					
Yes	9 (40.9)	5		10	
No	13 (59.1)	>50	0.001	>50	0.004
Skin or subcutaneous involvement					
Yes	10 (45.5)	6		9	
No	12 (54.5)	>50	0.009	36	0.012

TTP time to disease progression, *OS* overall survival
[a]These include three patients with a pathologic complete response

disease. Patients with N0–1 disease were excluded from the clinical trial, and 70% of the patients included had deep inguinal or pelvic lymph node enlargement (N3). Nearly half of them had skin ulceration. Disease-free survival of patients with these adverse features was historically 10–15%, and after neoadjuvant chemotherapy was 36.7%. Neoadjuvant paclitaxel, ifosfamide, and cisplatin is therefore a reasonable standard of care regimen for patients with bulky regional metastases.

Selection of High-Risk Patients

Assessing the bulk or stage of regional lymph nodes can pose a challenge. Much of the historical data on stage and prognosis was based on pathologic staging in patients who underwent lymph node dissection. In the 2010 revision of the AJCC staging system, extranodal extension was designated pN3 because it was associated with very poor survival [22]. These patients should ideally receive neoadjuvant chemotherapy, but how can extranodal extension be identified preoperatively? In a small series from The Netherlands, investigators measured the sensitivity and specificity of preoperative computed tomographic imaging in identifying high-risk disease (>3 lymph nodes involved and/or extranodal extension and/or pelvic lymph node metastasis) in patients who had undergone surgery [23]. Radiologists were able to identify high-risk nodal involvement according to the presence of irregular nodal border and/or central necrosis. This suggests that it may be possible to use radiographic findings such as these to select patients best suited for neoadjuvant systemic chemotherapy (Fig. 9.3).

Future Prospects

Targeted Therapy Based on Molecular Strategies in Penile Cancer

We anticipate that the future of multimodal therapy for penile cancer could include targeting of tumor molecular pathways with or without traditional chemotherapy combined with consolidative radiotherapy or surgery. Human papillomavirus (HPV) expression may be a reasonable method for stratifying patients [24, 25]; among a subset of penile cancers (29–56%), the biology of malignant transformation is thought to be driven by HPV. This could have important implications for progression as well as in the choice of and response to therapies. Among a group of patients receiving treatment for penile cancer at The Netherlands Cancer Institute, patients with HPV-positive tumors were noted to have relatively better survival [25], and that was an independent prognosticator of survival. In an analogous setting, HPV was a favorable prognostic finding among patients whose oropharyngeal squamous cancer was treated with chemoradiation [26]. After adjusting for prognostic factors, Ang and colleagues found that those patients with HPV-positive tumors had a 58% reduction in death [26]. Thus, future stratification of patients by this variable as well as identification of relevant downstream molecular targets will be important. In this regard, the retinoblastoma protein has been shown to be lost among high-risk HPV-positive cases, likely due to binding by the viral oncoprotein E7 [24].

Growth factor receptor targeting is another potential strategy for affecting penile cancer. Such receptors and their intracellular signal transduction pathways modulate cellular functions such as protein synthesis, cell turnover, cell adhesion and migration, and angiogenesis, among other processes. Several growth factor receptor inhibitors and tyrosine kinase inhibitors have been developed and entered the realm of clinical use in the past decade. Although there still have been no prospective studies in penile cancer, case reports have described responses to sorafenib [27], cetuximab alone or in combination with chemotherapy [28, 29], and panitumumab [30]. Zhu et al. [27] treated six patients with chemorefractory advanced metastatic penile cancer with either sorafenib or sunitinib and noted one patient with a partial response and four with stable disease. Three patients had significant pain reduction. These responses correlated with decreases in the serological marker squamous cell antigen

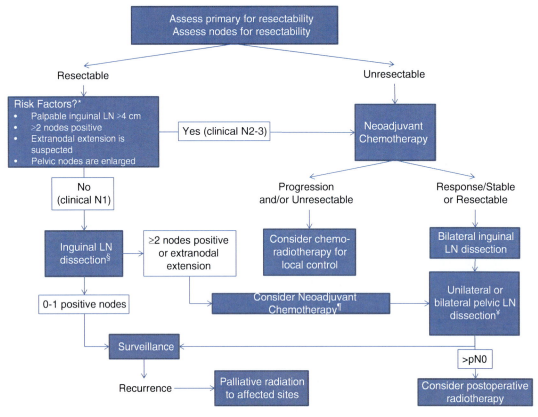

Fig. 9.3 Multimodal strategy for management of locally advanced and metastatic penile cancer. *Abbreviations*: *LN* lymph node. *Fine needle aspirate of suspicious lymph nodes is standard and can be used to identify high risk patients, e.g., bilateral inguinal lymph node involvement. §Superficial and deep inguinal lymph node dissection is standard on the involved side. A modified (superficial) inguinal lymph node dissection is recommended for the contralateral groin. An ipsilateral pelvic dissection can be performed on the clinically node positive side at the discretion of the treating surgeon. ¶Postoperative radiotherapy can be considered if an ipsilateral pelvic dissection was done at the first operation. ¥Pelvic lymph node dissection at the same time as inguinal lymph node dissection is recommended on the side(s) identified prior to neoadjuvant chemotherapy as high risk

and with decreases in microvessel density and proliferation, as judged by the results of Ki-67 staining of both pretreatment and posttreatment tumor biopsy specimens.

Further, we have studied epidermal growth factor (EGFR) expression and therapy among patients with metastatic penile cancer seen at MD Anderson [28, 31]. Thirteen cases were assayed for EGFR expression within tissue from lymph node metastasis in five patients, inguinal or scrotal skin metastasis in two patients, and from the primary tumor in six patients. Tumor cells in all cases were positive for EGFR, and all of the patients received one or more EGFR-targeted therapies including erlotinib (1 patient), cetuximab

(3 patients), or cetuximab combined with one or more cytotoxic agents (9 patients). Six patients received a second or third EGFR-targeted therapy. Grade 3 or 4 adverse events were limited to one case each of cellulitis, thrombocytopenia, and tumor hemorrhage. Two patients experienced disease progression during initial treatment with paclitaxel, ifosfamide, and cisplatin and then had partial responses to the same chemotherapy plus cetuximab. Two patients had partial responses to cetuximab and cisplatin, also following prior chemotherapy. Four patients (31%) survived 13 to more than 48 months, comparing favorably with their expected survival time. These results, although anecdotal, suggest that EGFR

is highly expressed in advanced penile cancer and is another promising target in our therapeutic armamentarium.

Future clinical trials should define the roles of these targeted therapeutic strategies among patients with lower disease burdens in the neoadjuvant setting either alone or combined with chemotherapy and subsequent consolidation with surgery and/or radiation. Defining molecular correlates of response and resistance to sequential or combination therapies should prove beneficial in enhancing survival.

International Clinical Trials

For clinical trials to move forward in this rare disease, multi-institutional collaborations will be essential. To date, as previously mentioned, there have been no randomized trials of multimodal therapy in penile cancer. To address this research gap, the US National Cancer Institute, Cancer Research United Kingdom, and the EORTC are co-sponsoring a collaborative group, the International Rare Cancers Initiative, to develop clinical trial concepts suitable for study patient accrual among international collaborators. If it is successful, such a collaborative endeavor will be a landmark event in the field and in the treatment of penile cancer patients.

Conclusion

Penile cancer with regional lymph node metastases is certainly amenable to multimodal therapy, in much the same way as squamous cell carcinoma at other sites such as the vulva and anal canal. There is now evidence from a prospective trial to support the recommendation of neoadjuvant paclitaxel, ifosfamide, and cisplatin chemotherapy in patients with N2–3 disease. We consider that to include any patient with three or more inguinal lymph nodes and/or pelvic lymph node enlargement and/or clinical suspicion of extranodal extension. Features that suggest extranodal extension include size (e.g., ≥4 cm), nonmobile, ulceration, or the appearance on imaging

of central necrosis and/or an irregular border. Chemoradiotherapy also has potential benefit but is not as well studied in this disease. However, with a better understanding of molecular pathways involved in penile cancer progression, along with regional and international collaboration, novel targeted therapeutic strategies will increasingly be evaluated in penile cancer to determine their potential efficacy.

References

1. Pettaway C, Pagliaro L, Theodore C, Haas G. Treatment of visceral or bulky/unresectable regional metastases of penile cancer. In: Pompeo A, Heyns CF, Abrams P, editors. Penile cancer. Montreal: Societe Internationale d'Urologie; 2009. p. 175–91.
2. Pagliaro LC, Crook J. Multimodality therapy in penile cancer: when and which treatments? World J Urol. 2009;27:221–5.
3. Skinner DG, Leadbetter WF, Kelley SB. The surgical management of squamous cell carcinoma of the penis. J Urol. 1972;107:273–7.
4. Johnson DE, Lo RK. Management of regional lymph nodes in penile carcinoma. Five-year results following therapeutic groin dissections. Urology. 1984;24:308–11.
5. Gerbaulet A, Lambin P. Radiation therapy of cancer of the penis. Indications, advantages, and pitfalls. Urol Clin North Am. 1992;19:325–32.
6. Ravi R, Chaturvedi HK, Sastry DV. Role of radiation therapy in the treatment of carcinoma of the penis. Br J Urol. 1994;74:646–51.
7. Flam M, John M, Pajak TF, Petrelli N, Myerson R, Doggett S, et al. Role of mitomycin in combination with fluorouracil and radiotherapy, and of salvage chemoradiation in the definitive nonsurgical treatment of epidermoid carcinoma of the anal canal: results of a phase III randomized intergroup study. J Clin Oncol. 1996;14:2527–39.
8. Vermorken JB, Remenar E, van Herpen C, Gorlia T, Mesia R, Degardin M, for the EORTC 24971/TAX 323 Study Group, et al. Cisplatin, fluorouracil, and docetaxel in unresectable head and neck cancer. N Engl J Med. 2007;357:1695–704.
9. Ravi R. Correlation between the extent of nodal involvement and survival following groin dissection for carcinoma of the penis. Br J Urol. 1993;72:817–9.
10. Lont AP, Kroon BK, Gallee MP, van Tinteren H, Moonen LM, Horenblas S. Pelvic lymph node dissection for penile carcinoma: extent of inguinal lymph node involvement as an indicator for pelvic lymph node involvement and survival. J Urol. 2007;177:947–52.
11. Haas GP, Blumenstein BA, Gagliano RG, Russell CA, Rivkin SE, Culkin DJ, et al. Cisplatin, methotrexate and bleomycin for the treatment of carcinoma of the

penis: a Southwest Oncology Group study. J Urol. 1999;161:1823–5.

12. Pizzocaro G, Piva L, Bandieramonte G, Tana S. Up-to-date management of carcinoma of the penis. Eur Urol. 1997;32:5–15.

13. Pizzocaro G, Algaba F, Horenblas S, Solsona E, Tana S, Van Der Poel H, et al. EAU penile cancer guidelines 2009. Eur Urol. 2010;57:1002–12.

14. Leijte JA, Kerst JM, Bais E, Antonini N, Horenblas S. Neoadjuvant chemotherapy in advanced penile carcinoma. Eur Urol. 2077;52:488–94.

15. Bermejo C, Busby JE, Spiess PE, Heller L, Pagliaro LC, Pettaway CA. Neoadjuvant chemotherapy followed by aggressive surgical consolidation for metastatic penile squamous cell carcinoma. J Urol. 2007;177:1335–8.

16. Pizzocaro G, Nicolai N, Milani A. Taxanes in combination with cisplatin and fluorouracil for advanced penile cancer: preliminary results. Eur Urol. 2009;55:546–51.

17. Green J, Kirwan J, Tierney J, Symonds P, Fresco L, Williams C, et al. Concomitant chemotherapy and radiation therapy for cancer of the uterine cervix. Cochrane Database Syst Rev. 2001;(4):CD002225.

18. Moore DH, Thomas GM, Montana GS, Saxer A, Gallup DG, Olt G. Preoperative chemoradiation for advanced vulvar cancer: a phase II study of the Gynecologic Oncology Group. Int J Radiat Oncol Biol Phys. 1998;42:79–85.

19. Montana GS, Thomas GM, Moore DH, Saxer A, Mangan CE, Lentz SS, et al. Preoperative chemoradiation for carcinoma of the vulva with N2/N3 nodes: a Gynecologic Oncology Group study. Int J Radiat Oncol Biol Phys. 2000;48:1007–13.

20. Theodore C, Skoneczna I, Bodrogi K, Leahy M, Kerst JM, Collette L, for the EORTC Genito-Urinary Tract Cancer Group, et al. A phase II multicentre study of irinotecan (CPT 11) in combination with cisplatin (CDDP) in metastatic or locally advanced penile carcinoma (EORTC PROTOCOL 30992). Ann Oncol. 2008;19:1304–7.

21. Pagliaro LC, Williams DL, Daliani D, Williams MB, Osai W, Kincaid M, et al. Neoadjuvant paclitaxel, ifosfamide, and cisplatin chemotherapy for metastatic penile cancer: a phase II study. J Clin Oncol. 2010;28:3851–7.

22. Edge SB, Byrd DR, Compton CC, Fritz AG, Greene FL, Trotti A, editors. AJCC cancer staging manual. 7th ed. New York: Springer; 2010.

23. Graafland NM, Teertstra HJ, Besnard AP, van Boven HH, Horenblas S. Identification of high risk pathological node positive penile carcinoma: value of preoperative computerized tomography imaging. J Urol. 2011;185:881–7.

24. Stankiewicz E, Prowse DM, Ktori E, Cuzick J, Ambrosine L, Zhang X, et al. The retinoblastoma protein/p16^{INK4A} pathway but not p53 is disrupted by human papillomavirus in penile squamous cell carcinoma. Histopathology. 2011;58:433–9.

25. Lont AP, Kroon BK, Horenblas S, Gallee MPW, Berkhof J, Meijer CJJM, et al. Presence of high-risk human papillomavirus DNA in penile carcinoma predicts favorable outcome in survival. Int J Cancer. 2006;119:1078–81.

26. Ang KK, Harris J, Wheeler R, Weber R, Rosenthal DI, Nguyen-Tân F, et al. Human papillomavirus and survival of patients with oropharyngeal cancer. N Engl J Med. 2010;363:24–35.

27. Zhu Y, Li H, Yao XD, Zhang SL, Zhang HL, Shi GH, et al. Feasibility and activity of sorafenib and sunitinib in advanced penile cancer: a preliminary report. Urol Int. 2010;85:334–40.

28. Pagliaro LC, Osai W, Tamboli P, Vakar-Lopez F, Pettaway CA. Epidermal growth factor receptor expression in and targeted therapy for metastatic squamous cell carcinoma of the penis. J Clin Oncol. 2007;25(18S):Abstract 14045.

29. Rescigno P, Matano E, Raimondo L, Mainolfi C, Federico P, Buonerba C, et al. Combination of docetaxel and cetuximab for penile cancer: a case report and literature review. Anticancer Drugs. 2012;23:573–7.

30. Necchi A, Nicolai N, Colecchia M, Catanzaro M, Torelli T, Piva L, et al. Proof of activity of anti-epidermal growth factor receptor-targeted therapy for relapsed squamous cell carcinoma of the penis. J Clin Oncol. 2011;29:e650–2.

31. Carthon BC, Pettaway CA, Pagliaro LC. Epidermal growth factor receptor (EGFR) targeted therapy in advanced metastatic squamous cell carcinoma (AMSCC) of the penis: updates and molecular analysis. J Clin Oncol. 2010;28(Suppl):Abstract e15022.

New Horizons in the Diagnosis, Treatment, and Prevention of Penile Cancer

10

C. Protzel and O.W. Hakenberg

Introduction

Many efforts have been made to improve the prognosis of what is often perceived to be the deadly diagnosis of cancer. In this regard, new strategies of diagnosis and treatment were developed within our rapidly evolving medical world. New therapeutic approaches have been developed based on the findings of large clinical trials, with evidence based guidelines created reflective of the data provided by these pivotal studies. There is a clear tendency and need for an individualized treatment approach integrating a patient's performance and tumor characteristics, as seen in novel therapies based on targeted therapies (e.g., in metastatic kidney cancer). Unfortunately, this extensive and rigorous scientific data is lacking for penile cancer. Reasons for this have been highlighted in preceding chapters. Nevertheless, there are centers of excellence in the care of penile cancer which have embraced international cooperation to improve the care and treatment outcomes of penile cancer. These chances are very much needed as we embark in a new era of medicine focused on a completely new level of understanding of cancer biology along with its inherent con-

sequences on our care of penile cancer patients which is the focus of this chapter.

To have a better understanding of the new horizons in penile cancer treatment approaches, we must reflect on the significant advances made for other similar phenotypic tumor types. A proper understanding of penile cancer carcinogenesis and tumor progression is critical for researchers and clinicians alike caring for such patients. Thereafter, we discuss new aspects in our understanding of carcinogenesis, tumor invasion, and metastasis which have emerged over the last two decades.

Important for future perspectives in penile cancer are four major points:
1. Tumor cells are different from normal cells.
2. Tumor cells include a special subgroup of cancer stem cells.
3. Metastatic cells are different from primary tumor cells.
4. The understanding of cancer mechanisms create new options for treatment but only caring for significant number of patients truly creates clinical experience.

Hallmarks of Cancer Which Create New Opportunities for Progress

Although the mechanisms of malignant transformation and dissemination are not well characterized, it appears obvious that human tumor pathogenesis is a multistep process. Cancer cells need to acquire capabilities that enable them to

C. Protzel, M.D., Ph.D. (✉) • O.W. Hakenberg M.D., Ph.D.
Department of Urology, University of Rostock,
E. Heydemann Str. 6, Rostock 18057, Germany
e-mail: chris.protzel@med.uni.rostock.de;
oliver.hakenberg@med.uni-rostock.de

Table 10.1 Hallmarks of cancer [1]

Hallmark capabilities
Resisting cell death
Reprogramming energy metabolism
Inducing angiogenesis
Sustaining proliferative signalling
Evading growth suppressors
Enabling replicative immortality
Avoiding immune destruction
Activating invasion
Enabling characteristics
Genome instability
Tumor promoting inflammation

survive, progress, and to spread into other organs. Hanahan and Weinberg outlined these capabilities and their respective mechanism in an outstanding article which they termed the Hallmarks of Cancer [1]. These hallmarks offer not only perspectives in understanding the disease, but have far reaching implications in cancer treatment. The mechanisms described in these hallmarks are shown in Table 10.1 and they constitute unique opportunities for cancer prevention, diagnosis, and optimized treatment of penile cancer.

Resisting Cell Death

The prevention of malignant transformation by apoptosis is one of the most important barriers to abnormal development and carcinogenesis in human cells. The apoptotic machinery is controlled by two different pathways, the intrinsic and extrinsic pathways [2]. The extrinsic pathway is activated by extracellular signals from cytotoxic cells in response to infection or other cell damage. This pathway is initiated by the receptors of the TNF superfamily (TRAIL, ApoL, TNFR1), activating the upstream regulators caspase 8 and 10 [2, 3]. The intrinsic pathway is activated in response to DNA damage and p53 activation. The upstream regulation of apoptosis is realized through members of the Bcl-2 family (pro-apoptotic, anti-apoptotic, and regulating proteins). p53 leads to an activation of Noxa and Puma which inhibit the anti-apoptotic effect of Bcl-2 and Bcl-XL. Bid and Bad activate Bax/Bak [2, 4]. Both pathways

activate the downstream effector caspases 3, 6, and 7 which initiate the apoptotic process [2].

Genetic alterations of both pathways are frequently found in tumor cells. Genetic instability is known for chromosome 8p21-22 (TNF receptors DR4 and 5) and for the caspases 8 and 10 [1]. Mutations and allelic loss in the p53 region are known for nearly every tumor type including penile cancer. While mutations seem to play a minor role in penile cancer, loss of heterozygosity is frequently found [5]. Mutations of p53 are associated with a stabilization of non-functional p53. Therefore, immunohistochemical (IHC) examinations show a strong expression of p53. Nevertheless, a clear differentiation between non-functional and functional p53 is not possible in IHC. As shown in previous chapters, strong expression of p53 seems to be associated with poor prognosis and the occurrence of lymph node metastasis in penile cancer [6]. Other studies were not able to show this association [5]. Although inactivation of p53 by HPV-E6 plays a key role in HPV oncogene associated carcinogenesis. Strong expression of p53 leads also to an inhibition of the cell cycle by the p21/ Retinoblastoma (Rb) cascade. This negative cell cycle regulation is also disturbed by HPV oncogenes, namely, E7, which binds and inactivates Rb (shown in Figs. 10.1 and 10.2b) [7]. HPV infection plays also a relevant role for carcinogenesis in basaloid penile carcinomas and in a relevant number of conventional penile carcinomas [8]. Therefore, HPV vaccination may play a possible role in the prevention of penile cancer in a similar fashion as in cervical cancer. One may argue that the low incidence of penile cancer and the uncertain association in 50% of cases may not justify the vaccination of all young males, but a relevant reduction of the HPV presence in the human population can contribute to a reduction of all HPV associated carcinomas (e.g., cervix cancer, head and neck squamous cell carcinomas).

Several attempts have been made to interact with the extrinsic and intrinsic apoptotic pathway in order to reactivate apoptosis within tumor cells. Monoclonal antibodies against the death receptors DR4 and DR5 (lexatumumab, apomab

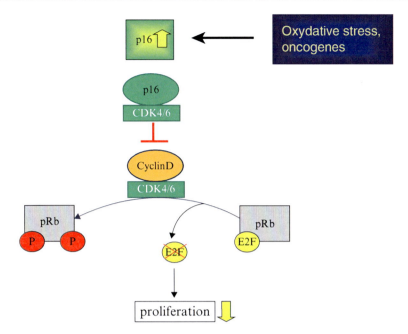

Fig. 10.1 The physiological role of the p16/pRb pathway in response to oxidative stress and oncogenes. The stress induced upregulation of p16 expression leads to an inhibition of the cyclin D—cyclin dependent kinase (CDK) complex, which is responsible for the hyperphosphorylation of pRb and release of E2F. E2F activates the expression of S phase progression genes. Therefore, p16 activation induces cell cycle arrest by blocking the cyclin D CDK mediated release of E2F. Modified from von Knebel Doeberitz M, Reuschenbach M, Schmidt D, Bergeron C. Biomarkers for cervical cancer screening: The role of p16(INK4a) to highlight transforming HPV infections. *Expert Rev Proteomics*. **9**: 149–163 [74]

and AMG655) were tested among the first clinical trials and showed antitumor activity as both single drugs and in combination with chemotherapy [9]. Since overexpression of Bcl-2 has been shown in several tumor entities Bcl-2 seems to be a possible target for cancer cell specific treatment. Gossypol and GX015-070 are both anti-apoptotic members of the Bcl-2 Family which have been assessed in phase I/II clinical trials. Antitumor activity has been reported for both acute myelogenous and chronic lymphocytic leukemia patients [10, 11]. Additional studies with the Bcl-2 antisense compound Oblimersen which is targeting the Bcl-2 mRNA have been conducted. A phase III trial showed improved clinical outcome and increased survival for the combination of Oblimersen and chemotherapy in patients with advanced melanomas [12]. In a small study, expression of Bcl-2 was demonstrated among penile carcinomas [13]. Therefore, analysis of Bcl-2 expression followed by clinical

trials seems like a reasonable treatment approach in penile cancer moving forward.

IAP inhibitors (e.g., Smac/DIABLO) were also tested in combination with chemotherapy and radiation in tumor cell lines. Other IAP inhibitors (survivin AS-ODN and Survivin siRNA) were tested in cell lines in combination with cisplatin based chemotherapy and showed chemosensitivity [9]. Therefore, these novel therapeutic strategies are all potential exciting avenues to pursue within our research armamentarium.

Reprograming Energy Metabolism

Permanent progression and cell division requires an adequate energy supply for tumor cell growth, division, and clonal proliferation. Therefore, the metabolism of tumor cells is characterized by special pathways first described by Otto Warburg [14]. Cancer cells change their

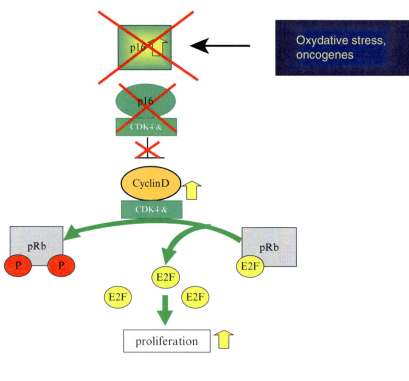

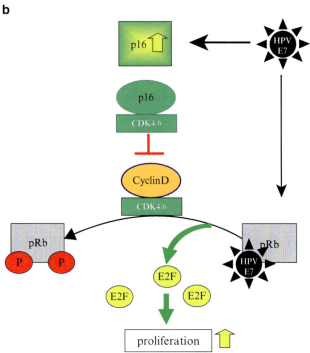

Fig. 10.2 Two ways of alterations of the p16/pRb pathway in penile cancer, resulting progression of tumor cells. (**a**) Promoter hypermethylation and/or LOH of p16 are leading to a loss of p16 function in the tumor cells. Therefore, the p16 mediated inhibition of cyclin D cdk activity in response to oxidative stress and oncogenes is lost. E2F mediated cell cycle progression is possible. (**b**) The HPV E7 oncogene induces an increased expression of p16. The cell cycle inhibiting effect of the p16/pRb pathway is blocked by E7 mediated inactivation of pRb. E2F is released uncontrolled resulting an uncontrolled activation of the cell cycle of the tumor cells. Modified from von Knebel Doeberitz M, Reuschenbach M, Schmidt D, Bergeron C. Biomarkers for cervical cancer screening: The role of p16(INK4a) to highlight transforming HPV infections. *Expert Rev Proteomics.* **9**: 149–163 [74]

glucose metabolism via a glycolysis pathway although there is sufficient oxygen. This process is called "aerobic glycolysis." The second important effect of this process is the diversion of glycolytic intermediates into biosynthesis of nucleosides, amino acids, and following macromolecules for cell division and tumor progression [15]. There is another tumor specific metabolic effect within the glucose pathway. While a part of the cancer cells secrete lactate by using the glucose depending pathway, a second cell type uses lactate as an energy source via citric acid [16]. The regulation of energy metabolism is influenced by activated oncogenes (e.g., *RAS*, *MYC*), by alterations of tumor suppressor genes (e.g., *VHL*, *p53*), and by hypoxia, which can all increase the levels of hypoxia inducible factors (HIF1α and HIF2α), both of which upregulate glycolysis and glucose uptake by upregulation of glucose transporters (GLUT1) [1]. The increased uptake of glucose into tumor cells is used for positron emissions tomography (PET). The ^{18}F-fluorodeoxyglucose (FDG) is used as a reporter for elevated glucose uptake which offers an unique opportunity for significant improvements in our diagnostic approach to penile cancer.

The detection of lymph node metastases is one of the most highly debated and controversial issues in penile cancer. While the sensitivity (87–90%) and specificity of palpable lymph nodes representing occult disease remains fairly accurate, the situation for patients without palpable inguinal adenopathy (cN0) potentially harboring micrometastatic disease remains challenging. Although the combination of a 40-row CT with a high resolution PET can detect lesions as small as 2 mm, the detection of single tumor cells or small tumor cell nests remains practically impossible [17].

Also, a novel application of PET-CT may lie in the evaluation of tumor response and prediction of outcome amongst advanced penile cancer patients treated with upfront systemic therapy. A key concept in this regard is the standard uptake value (SUV), which constitutes the FDG uptake by the tumor in a defined time period. For head and neck squamous cell carcinoma (HNSCC), a determination of SUV cut-off values for the evaluation of treatment response of lymph node metastasis allows to better predict the prognosis of a given patient [18]. A strong SUV decrease was associated with a better outcome. Another interesting aspect is a possible role of hypoxia specific non-FDG PET tracers in planning of therapeutic procedures. The ^{18}F-AZA and ^{18}F-FMISO have been used for the evaluation of lymph nodes in HNSCC patients. Patients with high hypoxia PET SUV (a sign of poor perfusion at sites of metastasis) received a higher dose of radio-chemotherapy [19]. This offers further options for penile cancer patients to predict the response to neoadjuvant systemic chemotherapy and targeted therapy by hypoxia specific tracers.

Another promising future option in targeting lymph node metastases in penile cancer is the hybrid fluorescent-radioactive tracer for sentinel node identification before inguinal lymphadenectomy [20].

Tumor Neoangiogenesis

Due to the extensive metabolism and growth of malignant tissue, an extraordinary supply of glucose and oxygen as well as evacuation of carbon dioxide is necessary. Therefore, angiogenetic regulators such as vascular endothelial growth factor receptor (VEGFR) are upregulated in most tumor tissues [1]. Angiogenesis is one of the major targets of systemic therapies for a host of tumor types such as metastatic kidney cancer. The role of angiogenesis remains still unclear in penile cancer, since there is no data pertaining to VEGFR expression within these penile cancer surgical specimens. Although a strong expression of angiogenesis-associated Annexin 2 was showed in penile carcinomas, the first attempts of targeted therapy with sunitinib and sorafenib showed only limited success in patients with advanced penile carcinomas [21, 22].

Nevertheless angiogenesis remains an interesting diagnostic and therapeutic target in penile carcinomas for the future. Perfusion analysis using multidetector computed tomography (MD-CT) allows determination of the microvascular density within tumors. Squamous cell carcinomas with a high vascular density showed better response to radiochemotherapy [23]. Therefore, evaluation of the predictive value of vascular density in lymph node metastasis may predict the response to neoadjuvant systemic chemotherapy among penile cancer patients.

Sustaining Proliferative Signalling

Detailed regulation of mitogenic signalling within normal tissue remains poorly characterized. Recent findings have evaluated several ways of sustaining proliferative signalling in cancer tissues [1, 24–26]. First, tumor cells are able to produces proliferation stimulators, i.e., growth factors and to express corresponding receptors to activate themselves in an autocrine manner. Second, cancer cells can also stimulate cells of the surrounding stroma tissue to secrete various growth factors. Third, a very important capability of tumor cells is their increased expression of growth factor receptors (e.g., EGFR). Fourth, tumor cells can also sustain growth factor independence by continuous activation of downstream pathways of the growth factor receptors. Activating mutations in B-Raf protein and in the catalytic subunit of the phosphoinositide 3-kinase (PI3K) are found in many tumor entities [1, 27, 28]. Another frequently found event is the disruption of the negative feedback mechanisms. These defects are able to enhance proliferative signalling as for example the loss-of-functions mutations of PTEN which leads to enhanced PI3K signalling.

Interaction with the proliferation mechanisms is one of the most promising aspects of new treatment options in penile cancer. One of the most frequently overexpressed growth receptors in various tumor entities is the epidermal growth factor receptor (EGFR). EGFR belongs to the group of ERBB receptor tyrosine kinases which also includes ERBB2-HER-2, ERBB3, and ERBB4. After binding of epidermal growth factor (EGF) or transforming growth factor α (TGFα) to the extracellular domain of the receptor, the intracellular tyrosine kinase unit is activated and induces several proliferative pathways within the cell which is supported by in vitro assays demonstrating overexpression of EGFR within penile carci-

nomas [29, 30]. Since treatment with monoclonal antibodies against EGFR resulted in a significant response in HNSCC tumor types, a targeted approach seems reasonable in penile cancer as well. The first promising results have been shown in recent single case studies for Panitumumab and Cetuximab [31, 32]. Since strong expression of EGFR has been reported to be associated with chemoresistance, a combination of classic taxan/cisplatin based chemotherapy with EGFR antibodies as shown for HNSCC seems also reasonable for penile cancer patients [33]. Current efforts are aimed on an international study for this combination in the neoadjuvant setting for penile cancer patients with palpable likely locally advanced/bulky inguinal lymph node metastases. Further development may be expected from EGFR specific tracers in diagnosis and treatment [34].

The Her-2/neu receptor also belongs to the ERBB family. Overexpression of Her-2/neu in association with aggressive behavior of the tumor cells has been described for breast cancer. Therefore, the antibody Trastuzumab is given in combination with taxane based chemotherapy in breast cancer patients [35]. Recent data suggest that HER3 and HER4 receptors play similarly an important role in penile cancer.

Inhibition of the PI3K pathway may be a compelling therapeutic target in penile cancer patients, since preclinical evaluation of PI3K/mTOR inhibitors showed activation in xenograft models [36]. There is recent data showing an activation of the PI3K/Akt pathway in non-melanoma skin cancer and Akt1 expression in penile cancer [37]. Further research is necessary to identify a possible role of PI3K in the progression of penile cancer.

Evading Growth Suppressors

Normal cells are protected by several growth suppressors which are activated in response to DNA damage, activation of oncogenes or exposure to mutagenic conditions. Tumor suppressor genes play an essential role in these processes particularly p53 and Rb are known to be central points of cell cycle control [1]. Loss of the activity of tumor suppressor genes lead to uncontrolled cell cycle activation by the cyclin dependent kinases (CdK). Another tumor suppressor gene closely related to Rb is p16. The tumor suppressor p16 inhibits Cdk4 and Cdk6 in reaction to DNA damage and oncogene activation (e.g., RAS) as shown in Fig. 10.1. Therefore, p16 is upregulated in response to Rb inactivation by HPV oncogene E7 [5]. Due to this association, p16 is used as a surrogate parameter for HPV infection in cervical cancer. In penile cancer, expression of p16 is frequently downregulated by genetic and epigenetic alterations (Fig. 10.2a) [5]. Therefore, p16 IHC is not useful for the diagnosis of HPV infection. Moreover, downregulation of p16 expression due to allelic loss and/or promoter hypermethylation led to a more aggressive behavior of tumor cells in penile cancer [5].

Inactivation of tumor suppressor genes by promoter hypermethylation is a frequent event in carcinogenesis and tumor progression. A significant increase in DNA methylation profile was found between non-invasive and invasive bladder cancer [38]. In addition to its prognostic relevance, hypermethylation is getting more and more enthusiasm as a possible target for therapy, called epigenomic targeted therapy. Treatment with azanucleoside is a possible way to rearrange the capabilities of tumor suppressor genes [39]. Therefore, further examination of the methylation status in penile cancer cells seems reasonable as a treatment strategy.

Another concept is therapy with Cdk inhibitors, which can suppress cell cycle activation [40]. The first clinical trials using such an approach have shown anticancer activity [40, 41].

Another tumor suppressor gene alterating factor, still in its infancy with regard to our understanding, is the activity of micro RNAs. These small RNA geness are processed after transcription by RNA polymerase II via pri-miRNA and pre-miRNA to mature miRNA [42]. Mature miRNA prevent its association with the RNA-induced silencing complex (RISC) by binding to the 3′-UTR of mRNAs. Recent data shows that miRNAs can also bind to promoter regions and stabilize mRNAs in case of cell activation [43]. Therefore, miRNAs can also activate or deactivate tumor suppressor genes. For instance, miRNA205

is silenced in several tumor entities [44, 45]. Re-expression of miRNA 205 by transfection of prostate cancer cell lines leads to cell arrest [44]. Apart of the tumor suppressing activity, it has been shown this interaction is mediated through the cell cycle regulator E2F1 [45]. Since miRNA expression is also frequently changed in HNSCC, further studies in penile cancer may help to identify its potential diagnostic and therapeutic role [46].

Enabling Replicative Immortality

The unlimited replicative potential of cancer cells is one of the most important factors for the sequential and often expansive growth of primary and metastatic cancer foci [1]. One remarkable limit in this process ought to be senescence which is usually initiated in cells after a number of cell cycle divisions have occurred. Thus, tumor cells have to overcome this phenomenon. Telomeres play a key role in the process of senescence. Telomeres are multiple tandem hexanucleotide repeats, which shorten progressively with each cell division in non-immortalized cells. The telomerase, a DNA polymerase, is able to add telomere repeats to the DNA. While telomerase activity is nearly absent in normal and premalignant cells, significant levels of telomerase are found in most malignant cancer types. Therefore, telomerase has become a target in cancer treatment in order to reestablish the regulatory mechanism of senescence within tumor cells [47]. Telomerase activity has already been shown to be present in penile carcinomas [48]. After further investigation, telomerase activity may become a target for penile cancer [49].

Avoiding Immune Destruction

The detailed interaction between the immune system, tumor cells, and metastasis is not yet known. The often discussed "immune-escape" capacity of tumor cells is underlined by the high number of virus associated malignomas in immune-compromised patients, including transplant patients suffering from penile cancer [1]. There is recent data showing tumor–host interactions in varying ways. Tumor cells seem to be able to disturb the immune system components by secreting transforming growth factor β (TGFβ) [50]. Additionally tumor cells may recruit inflammatory cells. Regulatory T cells and myeloid derived suppressor cells are able to suppress the function of cytotoxic T lymphocytes (CTL) [51]. This tumor-promoting inflammation seems to be another enabling characteristic of cancers. There is rising evidence that peritumoral inflammation plays an important role for tumor progression since inflammatory cells are able to produce mutagenic substances that promote genetic alterations in invading tumor cells [1].

On the other hand, there is evidence supporting the immunosuppressive activity of the primary tumor against the development of micrometastasis as well as for our innate immune response to certain human cancer types. The strong infiltration of colon tumors and ovarian tumors by CTLs and natural killer (NK) cells seems to be associated with a better prognosis for patients [52]. These findings were the impetus for several trials of immune stimulating therapy in advanced human cancers (e.g., kidney cancer). The role of immune-escape mechanisms and inflammation in penile cancer should be pursued in future research efforts pertaining to penile cancer.

Activating Invasion

The process of invasion and metastasis remains one of the essential characteristics of all cancer types, representing a multistep and multifunctional event. Cancer is also characterized by the invasion–metastasis cascade, which encompass interactions with the extracellular matrix in the epithelial–mesenchymal transition (EMT) program, invasion of normal tissue, followed by invasion of blood and lymphatic vessels (intravasation), circulation and survival within the bloodstream, extravasation and colonization to distant metastatic organs [1, 53].

Since tumor cells have to invade the lymphovascularity to result in metastases, clearly an unimodal approach of surgical therapy alone is clearly not enough in metastatic patients. Therefore, in every penile cancer patient with lymph node metastasis, systemic chemotherapy either in the pre-surgical or postsurgical setting has to be recommended [54].

The EMT program includes multiple morphological and functional changes in the tumor cells enabling invasion. Loss of cell adhesion and changes in the ECM are important steps in that process. Loss of E-cadherin is one of the earliest known changes with regards to cell adhesion molecules. Loss of E-cadherin was also described for penile carcinomas [55]. Low E-cadherin expression and high matrix metalloproteinase 9 (MMP9) expression were associated with a higher risk for lymph node metastases in penile cancer patients [55]. In contrast, other cell surface and cell adhesion molecules are upregulated. For instance, N-Cadherin, normally expressed only in mesenchymal cells during organogenesis, is associated with invasive growth and chemoresistance within cancer cells [1]. The changes in cell surface proteins during EMT are often most notably seen at the margins of the tumor. For penile cancer, a strong expression of Annexin 4 was shown especially in the invasion front of metastatic tumors [21]. The EMT process is under the control of transcriptional factors (e.g., SNAIL, TWIST, ZEB) which are normally regulated by metastasis suppressor genes [1]. The genetic instability in tumor cells, another enabling cancer characteristic, leads to allelic losses and mutations in metastasis suppressor genes followed by a loss of expression. For penile cancer, loss of expression of KAI1 and nm23H1 was shown to be associated with metastatic progression [56, 57].

miRNAs seem to play an important role in this regard as possible metastasis suppressing factors. In breast carcinoma, the cell lines miRNA 335 and miRNA 206 suppress metastases but do not influence carcinogenesis and of itself [58]. Both miRNAs suppressed invasion and migration in in vitro studies. In cancer cells, members of the miRNA 200 family inhibit ZEB 1 and ZEB 2 which inhibits the expression of E-cadherin [59]. Therefore, the expression of miRNAs 200 seems to be associated with a decreased tendency for invasion and metastasis [60].

The prognostic value of the expression of metastatic suppressors and miRNAs maybe potentially used to create future molecular nomograms predicting the risk of metastatic cancer dissemination. As we continue to debate the merits and drawbacks of inguinal lymphadenectomy among penile cancer patients, a marker panel such as this could be extremely useful in the future to better predict which patients are best suited for surgical resection based on the likelihood of having occult nodal metastases [61]. Particularly in patients with non-palpable inguinal lymph nodes, the loss of metastasis suppressor genes and miRNA would favor the necessity for an inguinal lymphadenectomy. Therefore, the analysis of miRNA expression is one of the major foci of penile cancer translational research in coming years.

This research should be also encouraged by the potential therapeutic role of metastasis suppressor genes and miRNA. It has been shown that treatment with cell-permeable nm23, as well as the re-expression of KAI1 after cell transfection, which are both lost in penile cancer, can lead to regression of lung metastasis within xenograft models [62, 63]. Lastly, miRNAs are discussed as potential direct targets or chemosensitizing drugs [64].

The Role of Cancer Stem Cells

There is strong evidence for an intratumoral heterogeneity of cancer cells. One special subclass of malignant cells are termed cancer stem cells (CSC). These cells are characterized by their ability to seed new tumors upon inoculation into recipient host mice [65]. These cells share characteristics with normal stem cells. During symmetric division, identical stem cells are generated whereas during asymmetric deterministic division, differentiated tumor cells are generated. A single CSC is able to create a new tumor with up to 10^7 tumor cells. Beside this main characteristic, the CSC show different expression profiles of biomarkers [66]. They have an unlimited potential of division. Since CSC divide not so often as normal tumor cells, they are more resistant against radiation and chemotherapy. A selective

Table 10.2 Cancer stem cell marker [73]

Tumor entity	Cancer stem cell marker
Head and neck SCC	ALDH1
	CD44
	BMI1
Colorectal carcinomas	CD133
	CD44
	Lgr5
Breast cancer	CD44
	ALDH1
	SOX2
	Twist
Melanoma	CD133
	ABCB5

elimination of CSC can therefore stop tumor growth [67].

The mechanism by which CSC are generated remains actively investigated. For HPV associated squamous cell carcinoma, a transformation of cells of the basal cell compartment has been described [68]. There is strong evidence that CSC are able to undergo EMT and are able to thereafter disseminate [69]. CSC are also found in metastases. Therefore, CSC are divided into local CSC and metastatic CSC [66].

Since CSC are able to escape antitumoral immune destruction and radiochemotherapy treatment approaches, they are suspected to constitute a major cause for local and distant cancer recurrence. Therefore, CSC should be one of the major targets of new therapeutic strategies.

As mentioned above, CSC are characterized by special biomarkers. They are different in several tumor types. An established biomarker for CSC in squamous cell carcinoma is the aldehyde dehydrogenase 1 (ALDH1) [70]. ALDH1 is involved in detoxification. It is able to generate retinol acid, important for cell proliferation and survival, from retinol [70]. Other CSC markers are shown in Table 10.2. These specific biomarkers are potential targets for CSC specific therapy. ALDH1 may be targeted by specific CD8+ T cells against epitopes of ALDH1. The strong expression of the biomarker BMI-1 might be another target for silencing gene expression by siRNA [71].

Until now, there is no data pertaining to CSC in penile cancer. Since chemoresistance and recurrence is frequently found in penile cancer, further exploratory studies pertaining to CSC in penile cancer should be devised.

Metastatic Cells

The process of metastatic spread includes not only EMT and invasion of stroma and vessels but also the seeding and mesenchymal-epithelial transition (MET) [1]. In SCC, this process seems to be associated with lymph node spread. Under special immunologic milieu conditions within the lymph nodes, cells are able to acquire further capabilities which enable them to disseminate into other lymph nodes or organs. In penile cancer, genetic instability is occurring during the invasion metastasis cascade. Examinations have shown an increasing allelic loss in lymph node metastasis compared to the corresponding primary tumors [72].

These adaptations enable the metastatic cells to invade other tissues (tissue-specific colonization).

Once again metastasis suppressors, which are able to prevent distant colonization (e.g., KAI1), have to be silenced before this can be initiated [56].

The differing genomic status and biological behavior of metastases, including the role played by CSC, demand a specific targeted therapeutic approach to metastases.

High Numbers of Patients Treated in Studies Create Evidence

Novel diagnostic and therapeutic approaches to penile cancer share the same problem. The number of patients treated in single centers is too low to generate large single center clinical trials and expertise. Recent collaborative efforts in Europe show the best way to overcome this major hurdle pertains to establishing centralized centers of expertise for such rare malignancies. The largest studies for penile cancer treatment originate from the Netherlands, where almost every penile cancer patient is treated at the university hospital of Amsterdam. Since this approach is not possible in bigger countries, the development of

Table 10.3 Future targets in penile cancer

	Hallmark	Target	Drug
Prevention	Resisting cell death	HPV alteration of p53/Rb	HPV vaccination
Diagnostics	Energy metabolism	HIF, Glut	PET-CT
	Angiogenesis	Tumor vessel density	Multidetector CT
Prognosis	Energy metabolism	Hypoxia specific tracers	PET-SUV
	Invasion, metastasis	(F^{18}-AZA, F^{18}-FMISO)	Expression of EMT suppressors (KAI-1, miRNAs)
		EMT	
Therapy	Resisting cell death	DR4, DR5	Lexatumumab, Apomab, AMG655
		Bcl-2	Oblimersen
		IAP	Survivin siRNA
	Proliferative signalling	EGFR	Panitumumab, Cetuximab
		PIK/Akt pathway	PI3K/mTOR inhibitors
	Evading growth suppressors	Promoter hypermethylation of tumor suppressors miRNAs	Epigenetic targeted therapy (Azanucleoside) Restoration of let-7 expression
	Replicative immortality	Telomerase	Telomerase inhibitors
	Invasion, metastasis	EMT	KAI1-, nm23H1 re-expression
		miRNAs	MiR-200c
	Cancer stem cells	CSC marker CSC specific miRNAs	CD8 T-cells against ALDH1, downregulation of BMI1 Overexpression of MiR34a

over-regional centers seems necessary and possible like is being demonstrated in the United Kingdom. Another approach has been adopted in Germany where similarly to what was conducted pertaining to the second opinion program for testicular cancer, a registry for all penile cancer patients has been established.

Since the number of advanced penile cancer patients undergoing systemic chemotherapy at any given center is low, the only way of establishing new systemic strategies in penile cancer is to design and promote international multicenter clinical trials.

Conclusion

The recent advances in cancer research bear great opportunities for an improvement in the prevention, early diagnosis, and treatment of penile cancer. Promising results of new approaches for other squamous cell carcinomas can likely be applied to penile cancer. The main targets of future research efforts are summarized in Table 10.3. New evidence based treatment strategies will likely parallel such international collaborative strategies and ultimately result in improved patient outcomes.

References

1. Hanahan D, Weinberg RA. Hallmarks of cancer: the next generation. Cell. 2011;144:646–74.
2. Ashkenazi A. Directing cancer cells to self-destruct with pro-apoptotic receptor agonists. Nat Rev Drug Discov. 2008;7:1001–12.
3. Peter ME, Krammer PH. The CD95(APO-1/Fas) DISC and beyond. Cell Death Differ. 2003;10:26–35.
4. Coultas L, Strasser A. The role of the Bcl-2 protein family in cancer. Semin Cancer Biol. 2003;13:115–23.
5. Poetsch M, Hemmerich M, Kakies C, et al. Alterations in the tumor suppressor gene p16(INK4A) are associated with aggressive behavior of penile carcinomas. Virchows Arch. 2011;458:221–9.
6. Lopes A, Bezerra AL, Pinto CA, Serrano SV, de Mell OC, Villa LL. p53 as a new prognostic factor for lymph node metastasis in penile carcinoma: analysis of 82 patients treated with amputation and bilateral lymphadenectomy. J Urol. 2002;168:81–6.
7. Sherr CJ. The Pezcoller lecture: cancer cell cycles revisited. Cancer Res. 2000;60:3689–95.
8. Rubin MA, Kleter B, Zhou M, et al. Detection and typing of human papillomavirus DNA in penile carcinoma: evidence for multiple independent pathways of penile carcinogenesis. Am J Pathol. 2001;159:1211–8.
9. Protzel C, Hakenberg OW. Emerging apoptosis agonists for bladder cancer. Expert Opin Emerg Drugs. 2009;14:607–18.
10. Tan ML, Ooi JP, Ismail N, Moad AI, Muhammad TS. Programmed cell death pathways and current antitumor targets. Pharm Res. 2009;26:1547–60.
11. Schimmer AD, O'Brien S, Kantarjian H, et al. A phase I study of the pan bcl-2 family inhibitor obatoclax mesylate in patients with advanced hematologic malignancies. Clin Cancer Res. 2008;14:8295–301.
12. Bedikian AY, Millward M, Pehamberger H, et al. Bcl-2 antisense (oblimersen sodium) plus dacarbazine in patients with advanced melanoma: the Oblimersen Melanoma Study Group. J Clin Oncol. 2006;24:4738–45.
13. Saeed S, Keehn CA, Khalil FK, Morgan MB. Immunohistochemical expression of Bax and Bcl-2 in penile carcinoma. Ann Clin Lab Sci. 2005;35:91–6.
14. Warburg O. On respiratory impairment in cancer cells. Science. 1956;124:269–70.
15. Vander Heiden MG, Cantley LC, Thompson CB. Understanding the Warburg effect: the metabolic requirements of cell proliferation. Science. 2009;324:1029–33.
16. Kennedy KM, Dewhirst MW. Tumor metabolism of lactate: the influence and therapeutic potential for MCT and CD147 regulation. Future Oncol. 2010;6:127–48.
17. Sadick M, Schoenberg SO, Hoermann K, Sadick H. [Current oncologic concepts and emerging techniques for imaging of head and neck squamous cell cancer]. Laryngorhinootologie. 2012;91 Suppl 1:S27–47.
18. Higgins KA, Hoang JK, Roach MC, et al. Analysis of pretreatment FDG-PET SUV parameters in head-and-neck cancer: tumor SUVmean has superior prognostic value. Int J Radiat Oncol Biol Phys. 2012;82:548–53.
19. Jansen JF, Schoder H, Lee NY, et al. Noninvasive assessment of tumor microenvironment using dynamic contrast-enhanced magnetic resonance imaging and 18 F-fluoromisonidazole positron emission tomography imaging in neck nodal metastases. Int J Radiat Oncol Biol Phys. 2010;77:1403–10.
20. Brouwer OR, Buckle T, Vermeeren L, et al. Comparing the hybrid fluorescent-radioactive tracer indocyanine green-99mTc-nanocolloid with 99mTc-nanocolloid for sentinel node identification: a validation study using lymphoscintigraphy and SPECT/CT. J Nucl Med. 2012;53(7):1034–40.
21. Protzel C, Richter M, Poetsch M, et al. The role of annexins I, II and IV in tumor development, progression and metastasis of human penile squamous cell carcinomas. World J Urol. 2011;29(3):393–8.
22. Zhu Y, Li H, Yao XD, et al. Feasibility and activity of sorafenib and sunitinib in advanced penile cancer: a preliminary report. Urol Int. 2010;85:334–40.

23. Faggioni L, Neri E, Cerri F, et al. 64-row MDCT perfusion of head and neck squamous cell carcinoma: technical feasibility and quantitative analysis of perfusion parameters. Eur Radiol. 2011;21:113–21.

24. Lemmon MA, Schlessinger J. Cell signaling by receptor tyrosine kinases. Cell. 2010;141:1117–34.

25. Witsch E, Sela M, Yarden Y. Roles for growth factors in cancer progression. Physiology (Bethesda). 2010;25:85–101.

26. Hynes NE, MacDonald G. ErbB receptors and signaling pathways in cancer. Curr Opin Cell Biol. 2009; 21:177–84.

27. Jiang BH, Liu LZ. PI3K/PTEN signaling in angiogenesis and tumorigenesis. Adv Cancer Res. 2009;102: 19–65.

28. Yuan TL, Cantley LC. PI3K pathway alterations in cancer: variations on a theme. Oncogene. 2008;27: 5497–510.

29. Borgermann C, Schmitz KJ, Sommer S, Rubben H, Krege S. [Characterization of the EGF receptor status in penile cancer: retrospective analysis of the course of the disease in 45 patients]. Urologe A. 2009;48(12): 1483–9.

30. Lavens N, Gupta R, Wood LA. EGFR overexpression in squamous cell carcinoma of the penis. Curr Oncol. 2010;17:4–6.

31. Necchi A, Nicolai N, Colecchia M, et al. Proof of activity of anti-epidermal growth factor receptor-targeted therapy for relapsed squamous cell carcinoma of the penis. J Clin Oncol. 2011;29:e650–2.

32. Rescigno P, Matano E, Raimondo L, et al. Combination of docetaxel and cetuximab for penile cancer: a case report and literature review. Anticancer Drugs. 2012;23:573–7.

33. Burtness B, Goldwasser MA, Flood W, Mattar B, Forastiere AA. Phase III randomized trial of cisplatin plus placebo compared with cisplatin plus cetuximab in metastatic/recurrent head and neck cancer: an Eastern Cooperative Oncology Group study. J Clin Oncol. 2005;23:8646–54.

34. Liu N, Li M, Li X, et al. PET-based biodistribution and radiation dosimetry of epidermal growth factor receptor-selective tracer 11C-PD153035 in humans. J Nucl Med. 2009;50:303–8.

35. Slamon DJ, Leyland-Jones B, Shak S, et al. Use of chemotherapy plus a monoclonal antibody against HER2 for metastatic breast cancer that overexpresses HER2. N Engl J Med. 2001;344:783–92.

36. Erlich RB, Kherrouche Z, Rickwood D, et al. Preclinical evaluation of dual PI3K-mTOR inhibitors and histone deacetylase inhibitors in head and neck squamous cell carcinoma. Br J Cancer. 2012;106: 107–15.

37. Stankiewicz E, Prowse DM, Ng M, et al. Alternative HER/PTEN/Akt pathway activation in HPV positive and negative penile carcinomas. PLoS One. 2011;6:e17517.

38. Wolff EM, Chihara Y, Pan F, et al. Unique DNA methylation patterns distinguish noninvasive and invasive urothelial cancers and establish an epigenetic field defect in premalignant tissue. Cancer Res. 2010;70: 8169–78.

39. Brueckner B, Kuck D, Lyko F. DNA methyltransferase inhibitors for cancer therapy. Cancer J. 2007;13:17–22.

40. Stone A, Sutherland RL, Musgrove EA. Inhibitors of cell cycle kinases: recent advances and future prospects as cancer therapeutics. Crit Rev Oncog. 2012;17: 175–98.

41. Luke JJ, D'Adamo DR, Dickson MA, et al. The cyclin-dependent kinase inhibitor flavopiridol potentiates Doxorubicin efficacy in advanced sarcomas: preclinical investigations and results of a phase I dose-escalation clinical trial. Clin Cancer Res. 2012; 18:2638–47.

42. Breving K, Esquela-Kerscher A. The complexities of microRNA regulation: mirandering around the rules. Int J Biochem Cell Biol. 2010;42:1316–29.

43. Dykxhoorn DM. MicroRNAs and metastasis: little RNAs go a long way. Cancer Res. 2010;70:6401–6.

44. Boll K, Reiche K, Kasack K, et al. MiR-130a, miR-203 and miR-205 jointly repress key oncogenic pathways and are downregulated in prostate carcinoma. Oncogene 2013; 32(3):277–85.

45. Piovan C, Palmieri D, Di Leva G, et al. Oncosuppressive role of p53-induced miR-205 in triple negative breast cancer. Mol Oncol. 2012;6(4):458–72.

46. Babu JM, Prathibha R, Jijith VS, Hariharan R, Pillai MR. A miR-centric view of head and neck cancers. Biochim Biophys Acta. 2011;1816:67–72.

47. de Souza Nascimento P, Alves G, Fiedler W. Telomerase inhibition by an siRNA directed against hTERT leads to telomere attrition in HT29 cells. Oncol Rep. 2006;16:423–8.

48. Alves G, Fiedler W, Guenther E, Nascimento P, Campos MM, Ornellas AA. Determination of telomerase activity in squamous cell carcinoma of the penis. Int J Oncol. 2001;18:67–70.

49. Buseman CM, Wright WE, Shay JW. Is telomerase a viable target in cancer? Mutat Res. 2012;730:90–7.

50. Shields JD, Kourtis IC, Tomei AA, Roberts JM, Swartz MA. Induction of lymphoid like stroma and immune escape by tumors that express the chemokine CCL21. Science. 2010;328:749–52.

51. Mougiakakos D, Choudhury A, Lladser A, Kiessling R, Johansson CC. Regulatory T cells in cancer. Adv Cancer Res. 2010;107:57–117.

52. Pages F, Galon J, Dieu-Nosjean MC, Tartour E, Sautes-Fridman C, Fridman WH. Immune infiltration in human tumors: a prognostic factor that should not be ignored. Oncogene. 2010;29:1093–102.

53. Talmadge JE, Fidler IJ. AACR centennial series: the biology of cancer metastasis: historical perspective. Cancer Res. 2010;70:5649–69.

54. Protzel C, Hakenberg OW. Chemotherapy in patients with penile carcinoma. Urol Int. 2009;82:1–7.

55. Campos RS, Lopes A, Guimaraes GC, Carvalho AL, Soares FA. E-cadherin, MMP-2, and MMP-9 as prognostic markers in penile cancer: analysis of 125 patients. Urology. 2006;67:797–802.

56. Protzel C, Kakies C, Kleist B, Poetsch M, Giebel J. Down-regulation of the metastasis suppressor protein KAI1/CD82 correlates with occurrence of metastasis, prognosis and presence of HPV DNA in human penile squamous cell carcinoma. Virchows Arch. 2008; 452:369–75.

57. Protzel C, Kakies C, Poetsch M, Giebel J, Wolf E, Hakenberg OW. Down-regulation of metastasis suppressor gene nm23-H1 correlates with the occurrence of metastases and poor prognosis in penile squamous cell carcinoma. J Urol. 2009;181:202.

58. Tavazoie SF, Alarcon C, Oskarsson T, et al. Endogenous human microRNAs that suppress breast cancer metastasis. Nature. 2008;451:147–52.

59. Korpal M, Lee ES, Hu G, Kang Y. The miR-200 family inhibits epithelial-mesenchymal transition and cancer cell migration by direct targeting of E-cadherin transcriptional repressors ZEB1 and ZEB2. J Biol Chem. 2008;283:14910–4.

60. Burk U, Schubert J, Wellner U, et al. A reciprocal repression between ZEB1 and members of the miR-200 family promotes EMT and invasion in cancer cells. EMBO Rep. 2008;9:582–9.

61. Protzel C, Alcaraz A, Horenblas S, Pizzocaro G, Zlotta A, Hakenberg OW. Lymphadenectomy in the surgical management of penile cancer. Eur Urol. 2009;55:1075–88.

62. Lim J, Jang G, Kang S, et al. Cell-permeable NM23 blocks the maintenance and progression of established pulmonary metastasis. Cancer Res. 2011;71:7216–25.

63. Takeda T, Hattori N, Tokuhara T, Nishimura Y, Yokoyama M, Miyake M. Adenoviral transduction of MRP-1/CD9 and KAI1/CD82 inhibits lymph node metastasis in orthotopic lung cancer model. Cancer Res. 2007;67:1744–9.

64. Di Leva G, Briskin D, Croce CM. MicroRNA in cancer: new hopes for antineoplastic chemotherapy. Ups J Med Sci. 2012;117:202–16.

65. Bonnet D, Dick JE. Human acute myeloid leukemia is organized as a hierarchy that originates from a primitive hematopoietic cell. Nat Med. 1997;3:730–7.

66. Dick JE. Stem cell concepts renew cancer research. Blood. 2008;112:4793–807.

67. Schatton T, Frank NY, Frank MH. Identification and targeting of cancer stem cells. Bioessays. 2009;31:1038–49.

68. Martens JE, Arends J, Van der Linden PJ, De Boer BA, Helmerhorst TJ. Cytokeratin 17 and p63 are markers of the HPV target cell, the cervical stem cell. Anticancer Res. 2004;24:771–5.

69. Chen C, Wei Y, Hummel M, et al. Evidence for epithelial-mesenchymal transition in cancer stem cells of head and neck squamous cell carcinoma. PLoS One. 2011;6:e16466.

70. Chen YC, Chen YW, Hsu HS, et al. Aldehyde dehydrogenase 1 is a putative marker for cancer stem cells in head and neck squamous cancer. Biochem Biophys Res Commun. 2009;385:307–13.

71. Chen YC, Chang CJ, Hsu HS, et al. Inhibition of tumorigenicity and enhancement of radiochemosensitivity in head and neck squamous cell cancer-derived ALDH1-positive cells by knockdown of Bmi-1. Oral Oncol. 2010;46:158–65.

72. Poetsch M, Schuart BJ, Schwesinger G, Kleist B, Protzel C. Screening of microsatellite markers in penile cancer reveals differences between metastatic and nonmetastatic carcinomas. Mod Pathol. 2007;20:1069–77.

73. Leal JA, Lleonart ME. MicroRNAs and cancer stem cells: therapeutic approaches and future perspectives. Cancer Lett 2012 Apr 30. [Epub ahead of print].

74. von Knebel Doeberitz M, Reuschenbach M, Schmidt D, Bergeron C. Biomarkers for cervical cancer screening: the role of p16(INK4a) to highlight transforming HPV infections. Expert Rev Proteomics. 2012;9:149–63.

Index

P.E. Spiess (ed.), *Penile Cancer: Diagnosis and Treatment*, Current Clinical Urology,
DOI 10.1007/978-1-62703-367-1, © Springer Science+Business Media New York 2013

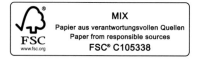

Printed by Books on Demand, Germany